HIDDEN IN THE BLOOD

BETWEEN MEN ~ BETWEEN WOMEN
Lesbian and Gay Studies
Lillian Faderman and Larry Gross, Editors

BETWEEN MEN ~ BETWEEN WOMEN

Lesbian and Gay Studies

Lillian Faderman and Larry Gross, Editors

Claudia Card, *Lesbian Choices*

John Clum, *Acting Gay: Male Homosexuality in Modern Drama*

Gary David Comstock, *Violence Against Lesbians and Gay Men*

Laura Doan, editor, *The Lesbian Postmodern*

Allen Ellenzweig, *The Homoerotic Photograph: Male Images from Durieu/Delacroix to Mapplethorpe*

Lillian Faderman, *Odd Girls and Twilight Lovers: A History of Lesbian Life in Twentieth-Century America*

Linda D. Garnets and Douglas C. Kimmel, editors, *Psychological Perspectives on Lesbian and Gay Male Experiences*

Richard D. Mohr, *Gays/Justice: A Study of Ethics, Society, and Law*

Sally Munt, editor, *New Lesbian Criticism: Literary and Cultural Readings*

Timothy F. Murphy and Suzanne Poirier, editors, *Writing AIDS: Gay Literature, Language, and Analysis*

Noreen O'Connor and Joanna Ryan, *Wild Desires and Mistaken Identities: Lesbianism and Psychoanalysis*

Judith Roof, *A Lure of Knowledge: Lesbian Sexuality and Theory*

Alan Sinfield, *The Wilde Century: Effeminacy, Oscar Wilde, and the Queer Moment*

Kath Weston, *Families We Choose: Lesbians, Gays, Kinship*

HIDDEN IN THE BLOOD

A Personal Investigation of AIDS *in the Yucatán*

Carter Wilson

Columbia University Press New York

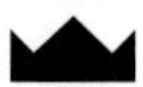

Columbia University Press
New York Chichester, West Sussex

Research travel was supported by faculty research funds granted by the University of California, Santa Cruz.

Library of Congress Cataloging-in-Publication Data

Wilson, Carter, 1941–
Hidden in the blood : a personal investigation of AIDS in the Yucatán / Carter Wilson.
p. cm. — (Between men—between women)
Includes bibliographical references.
ISBN 0–231–10190–2
1. AIDS (Disease)—Mexico—Mérida. I. Title. II. Series.
RA644.A25W59 1995
362.1'969792'0097265—dc20 94–23829
CIP

Casebound editions of Columbia University Press books are printed on permanent and durable acid-free paper.

Printed in the United States of America
c 10 9 8 7 6 5 4 3 2 1

BETWEEN MEN ~ BETWEEN WOMEN

Lesbian and Gay Studies

Between Men ~ Between Women is a forum for current lesbian and gay scholarship in the humanities and social sciences. The series includes both books that rest within specific traditional disciplines and are substantially about gay men, bisexuals, or lesbians and books that are interdisciplinary in ways that reveal new insights into gay, bisexual, or lesbian experience, transform traditional disciplinary methods in consequence of the perspectives that experience provides, or begin to establish lesbian and gay studies as a freestanding inquiry. Established to contribute to an increased understanding of lesbians, bisexuals, and gay men, the series also aims to provide through that understanding a wider comprehension of culture in general.

In memory of Roberto Crespi

Querido amigo, mas allá me voy morir.
[Dear friend, I'll die a little farther on.]
—song, "Querido Amigo"

CONTENTS

PREFACE

One night in the summer of 1987, as my lover and I were coming out of a popular basement club in Mexico City called El Taller (The Garage or Workshop), I happened to notice a single item about AIDS on a bulletin board. A newsprint two-sheet produced in San Francisco showing in photographs how to lubricate and place a rubber on a penis, it was the first piece of safe-sex information I had seen in Mexico. El Taller was a self-consciously hip recreation of a gringo gay disco bar with a cover charge too steep for many of the young men who might want to get in. But even among the educated middle-class patrons there, I had met very few whose English would be good enough for them to read the instructions.

At the time the North American press had reported little about AIDS in Mexico. I began asking friends who lived in Mexico City what they had seen in the papers there. Not much, they said, moral posturing from the Church and other elements on the Right, items about panic in smaller towns, young men who had returned home from abroad to die being driven out by terrified neighbors, but overall a sense of SIDA (AIDS) as a problem of the *extranjero*, of other places, not of Mexico.

My friends had also heard of there being some movement to organize among gay activists in the capital and in the north in Guadalajara. The federal government was preparing to launch safe-sex education campaigns, but so far none of the material had come out.

As in the United States and elsewhere, in Mexico the response of the government and the medical establishment to disquiet or outright fear generated by AIDS has been to "centralize" the problem for the popular imagination. You do this by assuring the public that a concerted *national* effort to "combat" AIDS has been organized, and that everything is therefore under control. In Mexico, that promised first prevention campaign was mounted by a newly established federal agency called CONASIDA, which soon had its own Harvard-educated director, its own journal, World Health Organization liaisons, research grant monies, and free information call-in numbers. Statistics on SIDA are now collected from all over the country, and the numbers are sent to the capital to be crunched and then published in a bulletin devoted to the subject.

But despite the effort to keep the *idea* of SIDA centrally contained, anyone who thought about it would conclude that SIDA itself was of course continuing to make its way into the towns and villages. I found it hard to imagine what the epidemic would look like when it did reach significant numbers of people in the provinces. Given how poor Mexico is—and its *increasing* poverty for the majority of its citizens in recent years—what kind of treatment and support could you expect to get for an inevitably expensive and complicated illness if you lived far from central?

By 1987 gay men and lesbians in the United States had already figured out that whatever various agencies of the state might promise, their own communities were going to have to provide the bulk of the education about AIDS prevention, and bear a critical share of the attention for those who fell ill as well. But in Mexico, outside the two largest cities, there seemed to be little tolerance for openly gay people and almost no political organization among homosexuals. Who, then, would take up the education and care-giving efforts?

Several people suggested I ask my questions at the offices of CONASIDA. But while I began to read the agency's materials as they were published, I resisted going this route. Policy concerning a crisis in public health is one thing, how people experience the crisis in everyday life can be something quite different. I was less concerned with the official version of the story than with finding out what I could on my own, starting more or less from scratch.

In the 1960s, just out of college, I had been taken on first as a student and then as an investigator in several anthropology projects in Chiapas. I lived in Indian towns and learned the rudiments of Tzotzil, one of the highland Mayan languages. I also paid extended visits to ethnographic projects in Yucatán and spent one winter in a house outside a fishing village on the Gulf coast there. I was always tempted by anthropology. I liked fieldwork, and the anthropologists I came to know practiced a kind of egalitarianism that made learning from them a happy experience. In the end I decided against getting a graduate degree in the discipline and stayed with writing instead. But the anthropologists had given me the basics of the old standard "ethnographic method"—observation, note-taking, interviews, participation—tools I still found very useful when I began to work on the question of how AIDS came to one corner of Mexico.

Yucatán seemed the right place to begin. Mérida, the capital, has grown to more than 800,000 and so is hardly a small town anymore (although its citizens complain that it still has a small-town mentality, everyone intent on knowing everyone else's business). The whole of the peninsula, which includes the states of Quintana Roo and Campeche, is now thoroughly plugged in to the rest of the world, both electronically and via the jet airports that bring the international tourists and take the local elite off to their shopping sprees in Miami and Houston and their pilgrimages to Rome. But modernization has been completely uneven and, in other ways, the Yucatán retains much of both its preferred isolation from the rest of the nation and its studied provinciality. Even in the heart of its cities Maya is widely spoken, and right beyond city limits Mayan rural culture still contends with (or rather, calmly proffers its alternative to) the lures of places like Cancún.

While I wanted to learn what I could about all aspects of SIDA in the *provincia*, my exploration also took the shape it did out of my being gay and wanting to get to know more about homosexual men in Mexican culture. Though I had not been "out" in any way in the time I spent in the Yucatán in the 1960s and 1970s, I had seen signs all around of some sort of sexual exchange among men, both Spanish speakers in Mérida and Mayans in the countryside. Now I learned that although male homosexuality is not much reported in the large anthropological literature of the peninsula, it is a commonplace both in Mexico and among homosexual travelers that the Yucatán—"white" and Indian—is a fairly gay place.

Ordinarily, I would probably have made a short reconnoiter of the territory and then would have arranged to spend an extended period of time in the Yucatán. But as it happened, four months before I had scheduled a first return visit to Mérida, my lover and I had ourselves tested for HIV (Human Immunodeficiency Virus). Ray's result was positive, mine negative. This stunning fact, which changed so much for us, also had its effect on the way I would go about working in Yucatán. Though Ray's health has remained fairly good, we now both have our reasons for not wanting to be away from each other for very long. So I tried to make shorter trips (a month, seventeen days) as productive as possible. By now there have been six of these—December 1988; March 1990; March, September, and December 1992 (this last one only a two-day drop-in as an added leg of a visit to another part of the country); and January–February 1994.

It was not until the visit to Mérida in March 1992 that I found a situation I knew I wanted to write about. Two years earlier I had met Alejandro Guerrero Flores, the director of the SIDA clinic at the Social Security hospital they call the "T-1." In the summer of 1991, when he came to California for a short training course on AIDS education, I introduced him to doctors and other people I knew in social service agencies concerned with AIDS in Santa Cruz. Getting ready to return to Mérida again, I called Alejandro and asked if I could observe the work of his clinic, which I had not visited before. I remember asking if I could be his shadow, follow along behind him "like a little dog." (The first of these images was echoed later when I heard Alejandro's assistant, José Manuel Polanco, explaining that in the office I was their *sombra*, or shadow.) What Alejandro arranged for me proved a wonderful opportunity, perhaps at times taxing for him, though he never said so, and further sweetened by the fact that through the time we spent together we were also becoming friends. I told him I might try to write about his work, and he agreed to that. When I had completed a first draft, I gave it to Alejandro for criticism, fully expecting that he might ask me to revise the whole manuscript. Instead, he corrected a few facts, but otherwise left completely alone what he calls my "novel."

The opening and closing chapters, "Those Out in Front" and "The Visitors from Wakax," take place mostly in and around the Oficina de Actividades Contra SIDA (Office of Activities Against AIDS) in the spring and early fall of 1992. What struck me most strongly was that Alejandro, his associate Dr. Russell Rodriguez, and their nurse assistant José Manuel Polanco were rendering a kind of treatment that, although not as high-tech as some in the United States, was remarkable in its use of the resources available (principally staff time) to preserve their HIV-positive clients' health as long as possible and to contribute to the maintenance of their dignity in very difficult, often undignified circumstances. As I say further on, the stereotype in the First World about the utter inadequacy, negligence, and inhumanity of Third-World medicine is partly perpetuated by our own medical establishment. It may seem a simple one, but a principal "finding" of this book is that clinics like Alejandro's exist.

Or, in the present instance, did exist. For there is no longer a separate SIDA clinic at the T-1, and much has changed there. So many people made me privy to the events of their often precarious lives that it has been hard to resist the temptation to continue to update their stories into 1993 and even 1994. New medications are being used, and the client load for Alejandro and Russell has grown. But except for a short postscript, I have kept to the form of an ethnography of a particular moment.

If the tale you tell is one that ends saying, in effect, "nothing gold can stay," your vision of the period at zenith should also contain a clear intimation of which forces of destruction are already at work. If I fail at this task, one reason is a lack of understanding of the vast federal bureaucracy of the Instituto Mexicano de Seguro Social (IMSS), which provides health care for up to 40 percent of citizens (primarily those with regular jobs and their families). It is not only at the T-1 that the SIDA clinic was shut down. The same thing has happened at other IMSS regional medical centers throughout the country.

The other factor I did not reckon properly at the time was the power of conservative thinking in the local medical establishment. Even before I learned that Yucatán has the largest per capita expenditure for health care of any state in Mexico, I was struck by the number of hospitals, the pages upon pages of private physician and clinic listings in the Mérida telephone directory. It makes sense, though. The city is a regional center, and for any health problems beyond the most basic, people can get there from all over the three-state area relatively quickly. But when they reach Mérida, they do not of course all receive the same level of attention. Viewed from another angle, the charming, hospitable city must be seen as the seat of an oligarchy of almost five centuries' duration. The ruling group, which traditionally drew its wealth from the exploitation of rural, mostly Mayan people, now maintain the upper hand through an ultimately stingy dispersement of such vital resources as education, nutrition, and health care. As researchers and practitioners, many members of the medical fraternity are up-to-date, but where social thinking on public health issues is required, they continue to uphold the old values of their class. Because the ideal unit in their ideology is still the monogamous heterosexual family, at least in the abstract they feel justified in denying assistance to anyone who deviates from the norm. In middle age, they profess complete ignorance of male homosexual practices, despite their own research indicating that sex between adolescent boys, or between schoolboys and grown men, is not uncommon in Mérida. On the other hand, they are tolerant of male *heterosexual* nonmonogamy, especially in themselves and their colleagues. When they come to make social policy, then, the paradoxes require them to engage in a variety of "strategic amnesia."

I would expect that the same story of foot-dragging and outright sabotage concerning AIDS is being enacted (with variations) by obstructionists in conservative local power structures throughout the world. But that means we can also hope that experiments like the one Alejandro and his colleagues mounted at the T-1 will continue coming into being as well.

The middle chapter of the book, "The Captain's Touch," contains three reports on other aspects of SIDA in the peninsula. The time perspective changes, enlarging somewhat. The first part, "Eddie's Nail Scissors," portrays several men I met in 1988 and 1990 and juxtaposes what they had to tell me about the homosexual "scene" and the arrival of the epidemic in Yucatán against the findings and opinions of the medical doctor who was the major researcher working on SIDA transmission at the time. The men were like me, middle-aged and middle class. They were also closeted and, though unwilling to be tested for VIH (HIV) disease, were deeply concerned about whether they had it or might contract it. Some of their bitterness and prejudice put me off, although I thought I knew their antecedents. It seems that in Mexico, as to the north, a knowing cynicism about all kinds of sex is one of the self-protective devices of homosexuals. The second part of the chapter, "In the Shade of the *Ya'ax Che*,"is about people who have come forward with help of various sorts in the face of the epidemic, including a Catholic priest whose moral support for homosexuals and understanding of the costs of social rejection I found singular, and the volunteers and clients at the nongovernmental SIDA group in Mérida, which is named after the Mayas' holy tree, the *ceiba* or *ya'ax che*.

The last of these three pieces attempts to pull together some of the scarce available information about sexual life in the Mayan towns of the peninsula. I concentrate on the even thinner evidence concerning sex between men, assuming that male homosexual behavior represents the first order of danger in terms of the spread of SIDA into lowland Maya life. Although sparked by several incidents from my trips to Yucatán in the 1960s and 1970s, the real site of this part of the book has been the library. Answers to the questions I ask here remain partial, which makes "The Captain's Touch" more a prospectus for a much larger investigation, one I would like to undertake myself or see completed by someone better equipped for it than I (someone, for example, who would not have to spend a lot of time learning Yucatec Maya).

Friar Diego de Landa, the man who smashed the Mayas' idols and burned their codices and then, back in Spain, wrote the *Relación de las cosas de Yucatan* (1566), the first great ethnography of the old ways, remarks on the people's hospitality to strangers. "No one enters their houses without being offered food and drink," he says. "If they have none, they seek it from a neighbor; if they unite together on the roads, all join in sharing even if they have little for their own need." What Landa wrote remains true in the present day. Many men and women in the Yucatán have been very generous to me with their time, including some who have very little of it to spare. I owe them all a great deal, starting with my debt to Alejandro Guerrero Flores. Because of the stigma of AIDS—and in some cases also because of the stigma of homosexuality—I have had to change some people's names. (In one case I have also changed the name of an entire town.) But whether they appear under their own names or not, I still thank everyone who makes an appearance in the text.

I have also received great help from a number of others, who have my sincere thanks. They include Victor Acosta M., Judith Aissen, Eric Ashworth, John Borrego, Nicholas F. Bunnin, Alfred Bush, Jay Cantor, Joseph M. Carrier, George Collier, Jane Collier, Barbara Crum, Candida Donadio, Monroe Engel, Rebecca Foster, Donald Frishmann, Jeffrey Escoffier, Jeanette Guerrero, Charlie Haas, Harry Harootunian, Melessa Hemler, Anthony Hixon, Robert M. Laughlin, Alan Lebowitz, Nan Levinson, Ray Martinez, Ann M. Miller, Jerome Neu, Linda Niemann, Daniel Niles, Sherry Phillips, Brian Pusser, Renato Rosaldo, Kristin Ross, Patricia Sanders, Carolyn Martin Shaw, Nancy Stoller, Jonathan Strong, Clark L. Taylor, Evon Z. Vogt, and Patricia Zavella.

HIDDEN IN THE BLOOD

THOSE OUT IN FRONT

MARCH 1992

Alejandro Guerrero works at two hospitals in Mérida. In the afternoon he usually comes back to the little house he rents on the west side of this sprawling tropical city for a short rest or some reading and a shower before going on to visit his second set of patients. The doctor lives down a dusty unpaved cul-de-sac in a separate apartment behind the home of a man who is an actor and theater director. On the ground level there is a living room with a wall of medical books, a kitchen with a gas stove, a sink, and a refrigerator, and a tiny *sitio* with a toilet. At the top of the outside stairs are a porch, a bedroom, and the shower. A metal stand in the kitchen holds bottled water, but the refrigerator is virtually bare and the ice cube trays have to be dug out of a formidable stronghold of frost. Alejandro has no phone. When there is a call for him in the main house, the landlord's little lap dogs come bustling out to the wrought-iron grill between the units, announcing the event before their master can.

While Alejandro is showering and changing, I read an article he has written for the in-house magazine of the medical center "El Fénix" in which he advises his colleagues about presenting symptoms that might lead them to test a patient for VIH. (Pronounced Bay-E-Ach-ay, *VIH* is the Spanish acronym for *Virus de la Inmunodeficiencia Humana;* SIDA is pronounced SEE-DA.) Many items in Alejandro's list of conditions that should put the physician on the alert are familiar—persistent generalized lymphoadenopathy, fungal lesions such as thrush (oral or vaginal) without other infection, chronic or recurrent herpes, rectal lesions in young men, unusual eruptions of herpes zoster in young people of either sex, tuberculosis of the lungs, weight loss, including weight loss in pregnant women. Other symptoms—like aseptic encephalopathy or meningoencephalitis, foliculitis, facial eczema, TB in other parts of the body, purple *trombocitopénica*, and *condylomatosis*—remind me of the vastness of the territory in which failures in the immune system lie hidden.

Alejandro is flying out tonight to a conference on AIDS/SIDA in Houston. Coming down from his shower, he invites me to stay here through the weekend while he's away. I thank him but decline, saying that at least for a few days I will stay at the hotel I've checked into downtown. Outside, the March sun is nearly down and it already feels a number of degrees cooler. We cross the street and walk a couple of blocks along Avenida Itzáes. Mérida has long been called *La Cuidad Blanca* (The White City) for the white-washed colonial buildings of its old center, the white *guayaberas*, pants, and even the whited shoes of the gentlemen, the pristine, sun-bleached *huipiles* with the bright embroidery at the neck worn by the *mestizas*, the collarless white shirts of the Mayan men. The broader streets of the expanded modern city, however, are planted with spreading trees that fill the spring with a showy succession of colors, currently pink *maquilis*, a domesticated Yucatán native, and blue *jacaranda*, to be followed by the extraordinary yellow cascades of *lluvia de oro*, and then the sharp crimson flames along the bare gray branches of the *flamboyan*.

ISSSTE—the Instituto Seguridad Social al Servicio de los Trabajadores del Estado—provides health care for federal employees throughout Mexico. Its Mérida center on Itzáes is a clean, spreading low-level structure that is used for administration and clinics, with a multistory hospital behind it. We pass down long corridors through now nearly empty connecting ground-floor buildings, Alejandro swinging his briefcase as he goes, and enter a large, bare examining room. It is chilly here; the air conditioning is working overtime. A nurse shuffles in, places a file on the metal desk, says she'll bring the lady, and goes out. Alejandro pushes two chairs in front of the desk, and then sits behind it. He offers me a chair, but I choose to lean against the examining table on the far side of the room. Alejandro takes a one-page report from his briefcase and scans it.

A woman and her eight-year-old daughter enter and sit. (I think the mother is about thirty-five, though I often underestimate adults' ages here by three or four years.) They have come from a city that is more than 130 miles away, not even in the state of Yucatán. I do not know how long they have been waiting to see the doctor. The girl sprawls in her chair. The mother has on a belted, knee-length imitation silk dress with a crossed-v bodice, made either at home or by a neighborhood seamstress. Pocketbook on her lap, ankles crossed, she leans forward, her hand resting on the corner of the desktop. Her daughter has been ill for more than six months—sore throat, respiratory problems, vomiting, and poor appetite. "Something like a flu that just won't go away," the mother says. And now this ongoing eye infection, which is the reason the case has been referred to Alejandro.

Alejandro's eyebrows are raised, as though in surprise or doubt. Listening, he sometimes looks down at the file before him, sometimes lets his gaze settle briefly on the squirming subject of inquiry herself. He is forty-four, hair graying, gray beard. The hair visible at the neck of his sports shirt is dead white. Despite tired smudgy circles under his eyes, Alejandro retains some of the aura of a reserved, high-strung, socially awkward but very intelligent student, the thoughtful one the other children turn to when they are in need of a plan.

The mother pauses, and Alejandro tells her that the result of the girl's test for VIH has come back negative. Showing no particular sign of relief, the mother nods and goes on listing her daughter's problems. Diarrhea, no taste even for foods she used to love—

Has the eye specialist sent the child to be seen by the neurologist here? No, the mother doesn't think so. Then, almost at once, Alejandro finds the neurologist's report right at the front of the file. When he mentions the doctor's name, the mother says, "Oh, him." Yes, they've seen him, too. She appraises her daughter critically and confides that on top of everything else, and even at this age, the little girl continues to wet her bed at night.

They leave. Alejandro packs up, and we make our way to the back of the building. "It's a *very* mysterious set of symptoms," he says. "Very little reason to think she might have SIDA, but it was a good idea to check anyway."

"Because of what? Toxoplasmosis? CMV retinitis?"

"Yes. Other possibilities, too."

We go through glass doors, Alejandro nods to a man in a blue uniform, and we pass into a waiting elevator. On the fourth floor the tiled hall is crowded with nurses, residents, chromed equipment. It is hot up here, so the doors into the rooms have been propped open. The supper hour is ending and families, wives and mothers, are visiting (children are not allowed on these wards). At the end of the right-hand hall, Alejandro pushes against the only closed door. His patient, a man named Jorge Alba Dzul, is the sole occupant of the large, four-bed room. Jorge is a thinned-out young fellow (I think twenty-four, maybe twenty-six) with tawny skin, a wide mouth, and big smoky eyes. His brother is also present. A stack of comic books and joke books with cartoon covers lie on Jorge's bed, which is cranked up to a sitting position, a metal IV drip stand at its head. Alejandro introduces me as an *investigador* from California, and both young men softly shake hands with me.

Jorge is in for sinusitis and a fever. Alejandro helps get his gown down off his shoulders and listens with a stethoscope, first at his chest and then at his back. Jorge voluntarily shows me the inside of his mouth, which is all white, covered with thrush, which Jorge calls *hongos* (fungi, also mushrooms). He wants to know how much longer he's going to have to be here. Alejandro says, "At least until Monday, so I can see you when I get back from Houston."

"What day is today?"

"Wednesday," Jorge's brother says.

Jorge turns back to Alejandro. "Monday in the morning?"

"No, in the evening."

Jorge then complains, though mildly enough. This room is stifling, but they won't let him keep the door open so a breeze could come through if there was one. He doesn't have any music and he'll go crazy if he has to be here all alone through the weekend. Alejandro asks Jorge's brother if he is going to be around. The brother says he will try to come. Alejandro promises Jorge he will write in the order for them to bring in a little radio for him and for his door to be left open.

At the other end of the hall is another closed door. Outside are lidded containers marked for contaminated refuse and a table with boxes of rubber gloves and paper masks. Alejandro twists and knots the two loose ends of the elasticized string before slipping both loops over his head and tugging the mask up to cover his nose and mouth, then helps me with mine, which has somehow gotten tangled in my glasses. He does not put on gloves. The room we enter is much smaller than Jorge's and cramped. It is occupied by two young men Alejandro introduces to me, Jacobo and Roberto. Their beds are against the walls, facing each other. A green-painted oxygen tank takes up much of the remaining space.

Jacobo has a sharp face, a knifelike nose, long hair that is damp with sweat. Jacobo is one of the longer-term patients, Alejandro points out, and he has been through a lot. "Any number of stays in the hospital." Jacobo nods, agreeing. He is a dance instructor in the town of Motul, an hour outside of Mérida.

Roberto comes from the other end of the peninsula, the Caribbean coast city of Chetumal on Mexico's border with Belize. Later, Alejandro tells me this patient arrived here just last week very ill with a respiratory problem that had not responded to treatment at the hospital where he works as a nurse. Roberto found out that his problem was pneumocystis pneumonia and that he had SIDA in succeeding moments. He has big eyes and a big smile, but he has lost a lot of weight in the last few weeks and looks exhausted. Beside him on his bed lie a big Bible with many colored ribbon markers in it and some religious comic books as well.

Alejandro inspects Jacobo's knobby feet, then briefly massages them. Jacobo says, "Doctor, I don't know what you can do, but I just find myself worried about everything all the time."

"What things, Jacobo? Financial problems?"

"That. Everything. Where money's going to come from, what's going to happen to my mother, what's going to become of my family, my brothers and sisters."

"Well, Jacobo, think about what good that can do. What are you in the hospital for? To get better, right?"

"Yes."

"So you have to concentrate on that. These other things can sort themselves out later. You know that. I'll have them give you something—"

"For my nerves—"

"Yes. But you've got to do the main work, which is not to get upset. I'm going to talk to your mother about this."

"You know she'll just get on me, Doctor, give me a *regañada.*"

"Well, then—"

A *regañada* can be a scolding or a reprimand, or something much more serious and humiliating, injurious to the recipient's pride or health.

Alejandro leaves the room briefly. Jacobo and Roberto ask whether I'm a medical doctor too, whether I'm going to Houston with Alejandro, how long he's going to be gone, whether this is my first visit to the Yucatán. I ask how old they are, then tell them I have been coming to the Yucatán off and on since before either of them was even born—twenty-nine years—which appears to please them. Alejandro returns and we get ready to leave. Jacobo and Roberto shake hands with me, say they hope I'll come back.

At a sink by the nurses' station Alejandro washes up with bar soap and the lukewarm water from the tap. When I ask if I should wash too, he says I may as well. In the elevator, as a kind of afterthought, he suddenly says, "In addition to the pneumonia, Roberto probably has a good deal of TB in his lungs."

Downstairs in the hall a little woman wearing a long white machine-embroidered *huipil* and carrying several plastic satchels stops us. It is Jacobo's mother. She is just on her way up to see him, she tells Alejandro.

"He's fretful today, Señora," the doctor says.

"Oh I know," she says. "That boy just worries about everything. And what does he think he can accomplish lying in his bed in the hospital? As soon as I can get up there I'm going to give him a good *regañada.*"

The son of a career Air Force officer and the eldest of five children, Alejandro was born and brought up in the D.F. (the *Distrito Federal*, or Mexico City). In his childhood the family lived in a series of rented houses in Coyoacán, none of them very far from the plaza, the bookstores, the cafes, and the park with the wrought-iron benches under the shade trees. One time I mentioned to Alejandro that on my stopover in the capital the previous day I had had a double pistachio cone at the ice cream store in his old neighborhood called *Siberia*. "Oh yes," Alejandro recalled, "where I used to take my little girlfriends when I was seven."

He was trained at the UNAM (the Universidad Nacional Autonoma Mexicana) and at the two Social Security medical centers in the D.F.—La Raza and the one now called Siglo XXI, which is just across from the French Cemetery, where Alejandro's grandfather happens to be interred. This particular *abuelo*, Alejandro's mother's father, had a post in the state government of Zacatecas during the Revolution, and at one point was pursued as far as the frontier and had to cross over into El Paso to escape. When victory came, he returned by train to settle in the capital ("those same trains in which the Revolution was fought," Alejandro points out). "At Siglo XXI many times on night duty I would stand and look out on the cemetery and think about him." Though eventually there came to be eleven grandchildren, Alejandro was the only one his grandfather lived long enough to see.

The revolutionary's grandson eventually chose tropical diseases as his specialty within infectious medicine. He was assigned to the Social Security hospital in Chetumal, and then as a *pasante* spent his year of required national service as the doctor for the Mayan village of Chunhuhub in the savannahs and the chicle forests of Quintana Roo. Before finally settling in Mérida in 1979, he also worked in Cancún and in Tuxtla Gutiérrez, the state capital of Chiapas.

The first time I met Alejandro, in Mérida in the spring of 1990, I mentioned I had spent some time in two Mayan communities in the Yucatán, but a good deal more up in the highland Tzotzil and Tzeltal towns of Chiapas. Almost immediately, Alejandro wondered if I happened to know Gertrudis Duby de Blom. "Trudy" Blom was a Swiss-born photographer, journalist, and crusader who had spent fifty years in the mountains and jungles of southern Mexico. I said yes, I had known Trudy since the sixties, and was pleased to count her as my friend.

"I have always wanted to get to meet her," Alejandro said. "She knew Diego Rivera, you know, and Leon Trotsky."

Alejandro's own discontent with things as they are manifested itself early. He took part in his first street protests before he was out of preparatory school. Then, in the months preceding the 1968 Mexico

City Olympics, like many thousands of others, Alejandro got swept up in the massive student movement that began to appear to have as its aim the overthrow of everything the regime of President Gustavo Díaz Ordaz and his predecessors had made of Mexico. Although an official in the Díaz Ordaz government, Alejandro's father was not opposed to the students or their demonstrations, which became increasingly raucous as the summer turned to autumn. There was no falling out between father and son, and Alejandro's father even allowed Alejandro's mother to attend some of the marches. Alejandro was present at the mass meeting at the Plaza de Tres Culturas in Tlatelolco on the afternoon of October 2 when, on a prearranged signal, plainclothes soldiers and agents of the secret police opened fire on the crowd. Alejandro and those he came with that day managed to avoid being submachine-gunned only by lying still among the bodies of their dead friends. They escaped the scene of the massacre and the mass arrests late in the evening under the cover of darkness and confusion. His father had warned them not to go that day. Alejandro assumes he must have known what was up.

Today, Alejandro remains close friends with other members of what is called the Generation of '68, including several who were imprisoned for years in Lecumberri, the so-called black palace of Mexican political justice in the D.F. The tapes Alejandro listens to in the evening are of the era—Beatles, Simon and Garfunkel, Aretha Franklin, The 5th Dimension. But in hindsight he criticizes the student movement for being too idealistic (or at least naive), and for having no base established with workers or other movements. When I argue that the students did, however, seem to have the approval of the majority of the citizens of the D.F., Alejandro agrees: "Yes, we did have that."

He recalls a filmmaking student who, as early as July 1968, stood up at one meeting and warned, "Every time we do something, the police react by doing something more violent." But no one paid any attention. After Tlatelolco, some of Alejandro's friends turned to Jesus or took other spiritual paths, and some became schizophrenic. A girl he knew just shut herself up in her room at home and wrote all over the walls, then painted them over and began writing again. At the end of the year, the young filmmaker killed himself.

"My generation," Alejandro says, "is like the child who grows up with the memory of having been beaten by his father."

Alejandro himself is a father of seven from four different unions. He delivered his own firstborn at the clinic in Chunhuhub and named him Canek, after the legendary leader of an eighteenth-century Mayan uprising against the whites. One son is called Inti, the Inca name for the sun, another Miguel Ángel, and there is a daughter named Aleida, after Che Guevara's second wife. Alejandro's youngest is a solemn, big-eared, three-year-old boy whose mother is a *Yucateca*.

From the ISSSTE hospital Alejandro and I walk in the twilight across the way to a private medical office where, since January, he has rented some space. A receptionist is still on duty and a couple of people are waiting, though neither of them for Alejandro. The office we enter belongs to someone else. I can pick out nothing of him in it. Although there is some air conditioning, Alejandro puts on a big electric fan and turns it in my direction. He sits behind the desk and smokes a Marlboro. "I don't have any clients," he says, laughing. "Well, a few. People who would rather pay for an appointment here than have to wait at either of the hospitals."

I have not seen Alejandro since last August when he came to California for a short course on mounting AIDS-education campaigns. At his little house he had mentioned the obvious—that he was living alone for a while. Now he informs me that he and his little boy's mother have split up. He returned from California at the end of the summer and found out that she'd been seeing an older man, an engineer. So he let her have the house and the car and moved out. The private practice was an idea he had for making some extra money. Now the engineer wants to move to another part of the country, so his wife has brought papers for Alejandro to sign so she can take their son away.

"It's been hard," he tells me, "through November and Christmas. But after the first of the year I began to feel better, less depressed." He laughs again. "I've even been going out some. Younger women, girls in their twenties. Not to sleep with. Just for talk, companionship. Because we get along together so well. Girls young enough to be my daughters." He shakes his head ruefully.

Saturday afternoon, the cooler bright weather continuing, Alejandro still in Houston, I stop on a downtown street and buy about a kilo of the tangerines they call *mandarinas*, then walk up toward the cab stand in Hidalgo Park.

Three gentlemen sit on a bench by their phone listening to the radio in one of their cars. I ask the driver who gets up and offers to take me if it is all right to sit in front. Fine with him, he says. He is an older man with his own wild, zigzagging route for getting through the narrow old streets out of downtown. As we roar along, he nods toward the back seat and tells me, "Yesterday, a customer got in there and put a gun to the back of my head."

"What'd you do?"

"I told him I'd take him anywhere he wanted to go."

"What happened?"

"He had me drive him around for a while, then he had me let him off."

"He didn't want your money?"

"It seems he didn't."

"Did you go to the police?"

"Why do that? If the man found out they were out looking for him, then he'd come looking for me, and he knows where I work."

The front of the ISSSTE hospital is all closed up. Along the street outside the side entrance people wait, leaning on cars. Up on the fourth floor I find Jorge Alba alone in his room. He is standing on a little metal step stool and leaning out the window. "My wife brought my little daughter to the hospital," he explains. "She wasn't allowed to come in, but I could see her and wave to her out the window."

"Don't let me interrupt you," I tell him.

"Oh no," Jorge says, "you're not. Her grandmother just now took her away. She'd been crying. She isn't really used to being away from home much."

We move away from the window. He is feeling much better, he says. Friday he had a high fever and sweated a lot, and he thinks that broke his sinusitis.

"Did you ever get a radio?"

"No, they never brought it. They said they don't have anything like that to give patients. And one of the doctors insisted on keeping the door closed and I had to fight him about that, point out to him that it was on my doctor's orders. So he finally permitted the door to stay open, but then he never came back in to see me."

I take out some of the tangerines I brought and put them on Jorge's bed table. "Do you like these?"

"Oh yes, I like them a lot."

"How are your *hongos*?"

"Still there." He opens his mouth and sticks out his pasty, gray-white encrusted tongue.

"But you can still eat these?"

"Oh yes."

A short young woman with long hair and lipstick comes in. "This is my wife," Jorge says, putting his arm around her. "Antonia." He introduces me as a doctor from the United States who is a friend of Dr. Guerrero. Antonia and I shake hands.

"What's your daughter's name?"

"We call her *Sha'il*," Jorge says.

"Is that Maya?"

"Yes."

"And how old is she?"

"Just two."

(I neglect to ask, and only much later learn that, in Maya, *sha'il* [or *X-Ha'il*] is a wildflower that blooms in the rainy season. Its colors are white, purple, and blue.)

At the other end of the hall, Jacobo and Roberto also look as though they are feeling better. The cooler weather is a big help, they say. Almost as soon as I arrive, Jacobo's mother comes hurrying in. Standing at the foot of her son's bed, she tells me that she is fifty-five, that she herself was just recently operated on and has barely recovered her own strength, that she has ten children and her youngest is a "Mongoloid," and that the priest they have in Motul is also a gringo, "and big like you, señor—"

"You mean with a big *panza* like mine, señora?" I pat my large belly.

"Oh—," she laughs. Their priest loves it in Motul, she says, loves nothing better than to go out to the coast and go fishing. They had another priest before, she tells me, from far away, but he must have been a German—

The conversation turns to food, and Jacobo and Robert manage to get in. They all like fish, agree on how good it is for you. Agree on how you have to keep up your nutrition. The food here in the hospital they think is OK. They only give you bread with your meal, no tortillas, but there is enough meat so you get your *proteina.*

Then on to the litany of the traditional Yucatec dishes. Does the doctor here like *cochinita pibil*? Jacobo's mother wants to know. Does he eat *panuchos* and *salbutes* or know about barbecuing shark with *achiote* and vinegar—

Yes to all the above, me nodding and tugging my little white beard, Jacobo answering for me, explaining to his mother that the doctor has been here many times before, off and on for almost thirty years—

Then Jacobo himself starts asking me about the dances. Have I seen them do the *Jarana*—where the men turn the little beer crates over and get up and dance on them? Yes, I say, I've seen that. And also men and women doing it with a tray of the little bottles of León Negro, called *chaparras*, balanced on their heads. And in turn I ask *him* if it's true what the Cubans claim, that the *Jarana* is just a poor imitation of their *Rhumba.* Oh no, says Jacobo, quite scholarly for a moment, the antecedent of the *Jarana* is clearly a dance from Aragon called the *Jota*, where they also put their arms up and the beat is three against four.

"Do you know how to do it?" he asks me.

"Not really," I say, "though I think I know the idea. I had a friend, Don Pablo Pantoja, who was a guide and a taxi driver, and Don Pablo always said—you'll excuse me, señora, for this—that the secret of the *Jarana* is that you have to be able to shake your hips without shaking your tits."

Laughter from the young men, a smile from the mother. "Well," Jacobo says then, "I hope you stay here long enough so I can get well and get out of here, and then I will teach you how to do it."

"Thank you," I say, "I hope so too."

From the center of town near the market, buses that run out northeast beyond the yellow railway station all list Clinica T-1 among the destinations painted in white on their windshields. Though "IMSS" and the name "EL FÉNIX" run in huge letters above the top floor of the three-story hospital building itself, no one ever seems to call the place "The Phoenix." It is "the T-1" (the Tay-Uno).

The main entrance is reached across a wide concrete plaza dominated by a large black statuary group on a pedestal. The fierce Mexican eagle spreads its strong wings to shelter the placid mother giving the infant on her lap suck from her full breast: the three of them together make up the often seen logo of the IMSS system, whose motto is "Health and Solidarity." Though thirty years old and conceived in a more heroic-democratic style, the T-1 has a basic layout which is like that of the ISSSTE hospital across town. On the ground floor, wide corridors surround open spaces planted with trees and lead to the consultation rooms and laboratories. Patients wait on benches or lines of chairs outside the doctors' doors. The administrative offices and the hospital itself are in a separate building behind the clinics. The T-1 is a "regional medical center" serving the states of Yucatán, Quintana Roo, and Campeche, the top or specialty tier in the three-level IMSS system. In the early morning there are so many people around that the place buzzes. By mid-afternoon, footsteps echo along the long dark hallways.

One of Alejandro's duties at the T-1 is to oversee and control disease internal to the hospital itself, principally the several varieties of staphylococcus infection. This is a job traditionally assigned to an infectious disease specialist. It requires many of the same skills needed to run internal affairs in a police department or to succeed as a confessor. "Bug doctor" is the name staff sometimes call them in the United States. An infectious disease doctor once told me: "In this job you always have to forgive people. Otherwise, the next time they screw up they'll hide it from you, which can only make things worse."

Alejandro's other chief responsibility at the T-1 is SIDA. He didn't come to SIDA, he says, it found him. In the second half of the 1980s he began to see an increasing number of referrals from other doctors puzzled by the appearance of diseases rare even for their latitude. (The three states of the *sureste*, or "southeast" of Mexico, all lie below the Tropic of Cancer.) The odd illnesses, of course, turned out to be opportunistic infections made possible by compromised immune systems. Alejandro came to assume charge of some extremely difficult multiple-problem and time-consuming cases. Many of his new patients were also people other doctors no longer cared to deal with for one reason or another. The other doctors were, however, often *very* interested in finding out who Dr. Guerrero's new patients were—so concerned, in fact, that they would sometimes come in and look through his files while Alejandro was out of the office.

Especially since what is called "The Crisis" of the Mexican economy in 1983, IMSS has suffered from budgetary problems, even in the face of increasing client demand. As a result the entire system has become, as the planners would say, "heavily impacted." For the individual eligible citizen, who is called a *vigente*, this all means longer and longer waits to see the doctor. For the physicians it means that, as Alejandro puts it, "at an IMSS hospital you have to accomplish everything very quickly." So, in order to concentrate his own energies, make things easier for his SIDA patients, and assure them a more confidential atmosphere, early in 1990 Alejandro got himself assigned coordinator of the T-1's "Office of Activities Against SIDA," which includes a clinical practice, VIH testing, and an education/prevention effort.

The unit occupies two large connecting rooms on the ground floor right inside the main entrance. Both rooms open onto the hallway, and beyond the second is a bathroom. There is no sign, but the glass on the front door is covered with a poster of the schematic version of the VIH virus, helmet-shaped, calibrated, indefatigable. Central but unobtrusive, the location encourages visitors, since the office is easy to find without having to ask a lot of directions. (One disadvantage would be that those seen going in lose the chance to take the VIH test, the *prueba*, completely confidentially.) In fact, all sorts of people drop in all the time, clients who are VIH-positive, friends of Alejandro and his nurse assistant José Manuel Polanco, staff members. Other doctors waiting to be picked up for lunch sometimes have their important calls forwarded down here.

José Manuel, Alejandro's assistant, is a bustling, chunky thirty-one-year-old native of Mérida. He and his boss sit across the room from each other at facing metal desks. José Manuel oversees the client files, which are lined up on two shelves right at his elbow, and answers the telephone. Neither of the phones in the room can call outside. (To do that, Alejandro has to go to the restaurant across the street and pay to use the phone by the cash register.) When people knock and poke their heads in, José Manuel usually leaps up, tugging his shirt down over his hips, and comes hurrying around to embrace them. Women friends he calls *amor* or *mi reina*, "my queen" (an echo of *mi rey*, "my king," which is what Mexican mothers traditionally call their little boys). VIH-positive clients often come in a little tentatively, since what they bring are problems or bad news about how they are feeling. José Manuel expresses delight at the sight of them anyway, chides them for not having come to see him sooner. "Have I gotten so ugly?" he says.

"Is that it?" He fishes in his drawer and, coming up with a blue plastic vanity mirror, bats his long lashes at his own reflection. "No, obviously not that," he says, putting the mirror away and turning back to the client. "You must have been on a trip or something, hm?"

José Manuel's exuberance, though fully natural, also includes its own element of calculation. As of March 1992 the unit has eighty-six clients from three states who are taking AZT (azidothymidine). They are given only one *frasco* (a hundred capsules) of the drug at a time, and since most of them take four or five capsules a day, they have to come in for their refills about every three weeks. Some clients have to travel five or six hours by bus or car to get to Mérida, but this way Alejandro can be sure that their progress is monitored regularly. For his part, José Manuel is quite aware that running a friendly, encouraging operation helps to keep the clients coming in.

Though Alejandro agrees, he says sometimes the atmosphere puts off heterosexual clients. When he can't get the privacy he needs for a serious talk with someone who is VIH-positive, he will take the client across the street for a cup of coffee. And with all the coming and going, he sometimes finds it hard to concentrate on his own work. But instead of moving into the largely unused back room for more privacy, he turns on the radio he keeps by his desk.

José Manuel has worked with Alejandro for more than two years. In exchange for his complete devotion, he is sometimes allowed to take enormous liberties with his boss. Alejandro asks José Manuel to go into his files and get a particular piece of information from every case. "Living *and* deceased?" "Both." This means looking into almost two hundred folders. "And when does the *jefe* want all this?" "Today. Tomorrow at the latest." So José Manuel calls Alejandro a "slave driver," but the next afternoon the figures are ready. The assistant also monitors his chief's social life. Knowing that Alejandro has a date, José Manuel asks if there is going to be anything more to it, and Alejandro says he thinks probably not. "Just supper." The next morning when Alejandro comes in to work all showered and shaved and whistling, José Manuel says, "I note, Doctor, that there was supper and *then* there was dessert."

Free VIH testing is offered every morning from seven to nine. José Manuel draws the blood at a round table in the center of the room and the following working day informs the client of the result. This means, on average, that every week he has the duty of informing a couple of people—many of them his friends—that they are positive for VIH. The hours for the testing are early because of the T-1's lab, which wants its blood in the morning. Until 1991, positive Elisa samples had to be sent off for confirmation by the Western Blot test, but now, through what Alejandro calls "our triumph, worth emulating," a chemist was sent to be trained at La Raza in Mexico City, so the Western Blot is also run at the T-1.

The other SIDA doctor at the hospital is Russell Rodriguez Sánchez, an immunologist also trained in internal medicine and infectious disease. Russell has taken over major clinic and in-patient responsibilities, leaving Alejandro more time to tilt with the bureaucracy and try to keep a research record of what is happening to their clients. Russell is forty-one, married to a doctor, the father of a son and daughter. He has curly hair that peaks in front, a mustache, sharp dark eyes. When he is thinking, he has the habit of tugging his lower lip way out, then letting it go. Under his white doctor's coat he wears silk neckties and white or pale blue dress shirts, some of which are frayed at the collar. Russell's father was Cuban, but his mother is a native *Yucateca*. Though Russell knows some English, he doesn't use it very much except for joking. Alejandro always introduces me as Carter, but Russell also notices that I sometimes refer to myself as Carlos, so he opts for calling me Charlie.

Monday morning. Alejandro, just back from Houston, is telling Russell how, on Saturday, I just walked into the ISSSTE hospital and went right up to visit his fourth-floor patients.

Russell looks at me. "You didn't have a pass or anything, Charlie?"

"No."

"And they just let you in?"

"They asked me who I was coming to see, so I named one of the guys."

Russell shakes his head.

Alejandro says, "Here, I'm going to take Carter up to meet the director and tell him we want him to have access to everything. Do you see any objections?"

"You'll find out, won't you?" Russell says.

Alejandro calls for an appointment and we are told to come at eleven. When the hour arrives, Alejandro goes into the bathroom and combs his hair, and we go over to the three-story structure. In a big outer office the secretaries all know Alejandro. They tell us to go right in.

The director, Dr. Ivan Aguilar, is fairly new to his appointment, a pediatrician with curly white hair and a mild, pleasant manner. (The manner turns out to be somewhat deceptive, since Dr. Aguilar proves to be quite acute.) We shake hands. The director asks Alejandro how Houston was. Alejandro says he will have a written report later in the day. We sit.

Alejandro makes a little speech: He and I have known each other for two years. Professor Wilson is an investigator in social sciences at the University of California with a background in anthropology. He speaks Tzotzil, one of the Mayan languages of Chiapas, and he has spent time here in Yucatán, in the town of Ticul and out on the coast in the fishing village of Chelem. He is interested in finding out what is happening to the Maya here with regard to SIDA. Alejandro tells how I was helpful to him when he was at the training program in Santa Cruz last summer and mentions we have put in for a cooperative research and training grant through a University of California group called MEXUS. "I have spoken with Russell," Alejandro concludes, "and while Carter is here we would like him to be able to observe everything we are doing."

"Such as?"

"For example, to go on the wards with us—" The director continues looking me over and nodding pleasantly. Then it is my turn to make a short speech. In my nervousness, I also hit on the pleasure of getting to know Alejandro and on the joys of collaboration, and my Spanish doesn't come the way I would like it to.

Dr. Aguilar waits for me, then rather abruptly turns to the question of the liability of doctors who infect their patients. He knows the story of Kimberly Bergalis, the young woman in Florida who claimed she contracted AIDS from her dentist, and about the surgeon at San Francisco General who gave up operating there because she thought the HIV risk to herself was too great.

Then suddenly the meeting is over. We shake hands, the director welcomes me, we are out and down the hall. I feel I've performed poorly and have to ask Alejandro whether he got the authorizations.

"Everything I asked for," he says.

The door to the SIDA office is propped open because the air conditioning unit high in the rear wall has chosen this morning to conk out. José Manuel heats water for instant coffee in a ceramic pot with an electric coil on a small table beside his desk. Russell, on a break from his morning office hours at the other end of the building, skims the *Diario de Yucatán* while he waits for his coffee. A technician in "whites" and white tennis shoes comes in, shakes Russell's hand, and begins a series of questions: "Doctor, what's the story? If one of your patient's blood goes on the floor, how dangerous is that? Do you have to wear gloves to clean it up? How long does this thing live outside the body? But a needle stick is more dangerous, right?"

Then in comes Jenny, a thin, pretty, and very pregnant young woman in a pink dress. Jenny spends a few hours each day at her own little desk in the back of the room doing the unit's typing. It seems hard to believe that she possesses the force needed to make the big sticky manual machine thwomp out the letters, but she does.

"Isn't it somebody's birthday this week?" José Manuel asks as he starts passing around the coffee.

Jenny admits it's hers, on Saturday.

Then we should have cake, the men of the office say. Friday. No, Friday Jenny has the day off. Thursday, then, they agree—we'll have a little celebration Thursday when you get here, Jenny.

Two young people come in, a couple. Both in pants, both with cheap tote bags over their shoulders. Middle twenties. The woman is pretty, made up. As she sits listening to José Manuel, her long brown hair tumbles forward and her knees jump up and down. She and her husband have both tested positive. They work in one of the new resort towns out on the Caribbean coast and have just arrived here on their way to Mexico City, where both are going to take the T helper cell test for the first time.

They move across the room to Alejandro, who uses Jenny's typewriter to complete their forms. The wife is three months and three weeks pregnant. It is her second *embarazo*. The first one aborted naturally. Alejandro asks how that happened. She had a high fever, she says, and then she lost the baby. As she waits for the doctor to finish typing something, her fingers play along her thigh.

Alejandro pauses, looks at what he has just written. I assume he is about to ask the woman if she thinks she miscarried the first time because she was seropositive then, but he doesn't.

The husband hasn't had any symptoms yet.

The wife claims no other sexual experience outside her marriage. The young man says he was in three other relationships (*parejas*) before they got together. Alejandro asks has he had any experiences with men, and he says no he hasn't.

Alejandro doesn't push. I have the feeling if there were more privacy here, if I weren't present, or if Alejandro or José Manuel were alone with either of them, other information might emerge. Today, however, is only their second or third visit to this clinic, and the question of how they became infected is not pursued.

They move back to José Manuel, who asks them to listen carefully. The hospital here will get them vouchers for their bus tickets to Mexico City (eighteen hours travel time each way on the express), and for their hotel there. Do they know the D.F.? They say they do. Good. They should plan, then, to appear early next Monday morning at the Hospital La Raza. Do they know where that is? It's also the name of the Metro stop. A particular form, which is extremely important, will be given to them. José Manuel hunts up an example from someone else's file. They *must* take the form they are given with them to La Raza or else they will not be allowed to take the test. Then they wait overnight, and the next morning the results will be ready and they can bring them back here with them.

José Manuel explains everything very carefully, like a parent giving instructions to children. Though the young people sit close, heads down, nodding and agreeing to everything, they seem isolated from each other. Getting up to go, they collect their tote bags, thank José Manuel and Alejandro, then the man opens the door for the woman and she precedes him out into the busy hall.

Alejandro knows a woman, a professional from an upper-class family with connections in national politics, a widow nearly finished raising two daughters. Many of the woman's friends are gay, Alejandro says, and they have convinced her that half the men in Yucatán are bisexual. Now, whenever she meets a man she finds interesting, she goes immediately to her gay friends to get the gossip on what the man's sexual life has been like.

Mexico approaches 10,000 cases of SIDA reported, living and dead, at the same moment the city of San Francisco approaches 10,000 deaths from the disease. But Mexico ranks third in the hemisphere in the incidence of the disease, following the United States and Brazil. The three states of the *sureste* have accounted for 4 percent of the national figure (about 250 cases), which puts the region right on the average for Mexico. Alejandro's clinic at the T-1 has dealt with 190 of the 250 cases. More than 40 percent of these have occurred in what Alejandro calls "heterosexual situations." By this he means that the infection appears in heterosexually identified men, in their wives or regular female partners, and, by way of intrauterine (vertical) transmission, in their newborn children. A ninth of people with VIH disease in Mexico are now women. In the Yucatán peninsula, the figure is slightly higher, closer to one-eighth.

Forty-four percent of Alejandro's clients at the T-1 describe themselves as homosexual, 32 percent say they are bisexual, and 12 percent heterosexual. These are all men. Women patients (also 12 percent) have all been presumed to be heterosexual.

The first anthropological study of male homosexual behavior in Mexico was begun by Joseph Carrier in the city of Guadalajara in the late 1960s. In his Ph.D. thesis, finished in 1972, and an influential series of articles, Carrier develops the idea that in Mexico the critical distinction is not whether a man engages in sex with other men, but whether he is "active" or "passive" ("insertor" or "insertee") in anal intercourse. Whatever his feelings for the men he has sex with, an *activo* is free to maintain the image of himself as a (heterosexual) "man." He retains all the considerable privilege due him in a *machista* or "masculinist" society. Unlike his gringo counterpart, he need not fear that one homosexual contact or discovering feelings of attraction to another man will make him forever "queer." Using Carrier's perceptions, sociologist Tomás Almaguér points out the important difference in the theories of the two cultures: in gringo society sexual identity is determined by sexual activity (any homosexual performance or even the homosexual thought make one "a homosexual"); in Mexico, at least theoretically, as long as a man remains "on top" in the act, nothing he can do (or think) can detract from his "manliness." The sex of the object of a man's desire, critical to the Anglo-Saxon, is in some way irrelevant to the Latin.

The theorists also point out that the construction of Mexican straight male sexuality depends on the sexual object being somehow a lesser thing. A man who is *pasivo* in anal intercourse is "no better than a woman," and may be thought of or treated as one. In street terms, he is a *puto* (defined in the dictionary as a "sodomite"; the feminine form, *puta*, means of course "prostitute") or a *maricón* (queer) or, in the south of Mexico, a *mampo*, which elsewhere is a black person. Asked if he is a *homosexual*, he is likely to answer yes. But the man he is having sex with regularly may answer no to the same question, and may also be offended by the question.

In his Guadalajara interviews, Carrier found that many men had begun homosexual activity in childhood or in early adolescence with neighbor boys or members of their own extended families, with older relatives (cousins, uncles), or adult neighbors. One theory in this regard is that traditional upbringing and Catholic morality keep adolescent boys and girls from opportunities to have sex, so the males engage in anal intercourse with each other as "compensation." Joe Carrier records cases where the relationship between young men who have been lovers in adolescence continues in secret—or even with the wife's knowledge—long after one or both men have married.

A principal reason given for why Mexican adult male bisexuality is so widespread is the "cultural centrality of the family." The idea is that the strength of traditional social patterns make it *unthinkable* for most men not to marry and father children. So desire for sex (or intimacy) with other men is made to accommodate to the prevailing custom. (Although usually not bragged about, casual sex or even an extended affair with another man fits easily within the code of manliness as a variant form of the extramarital *aventura*, which is often taken to be a husband's right in Mexico.) Even the rigid division of home versus work duties by sex lends support to the family as an institution. Men are not supposed to be competent to navigate daily life by themselves. They seldom learn how to cook or keep house and rarely leave home to set up a separate residence before they marry. For a man to continue living with his parents into middle age or to care for his widowed mother is not necessarily a cause for tongues to wag about his sex life. A Mexican psychiatrist friend once told me, "The big difference between our countries is that here it is still OK to worship the mother."

The Mexican men who describe themselves as gay are mostly middle- or upper-class, educated, urban people with exposure to international culture. Some of them are so sophisticated that they reject the terms *gay* and *apoyo gay* (gay pride) as imports, concepts not appropriate to what they call "Mexican reality." Some fear that forcing people to declare themselves will destroy the delicious existing ambiguous twilight atmosphere where all men are still at least potentially available to other men. (The international gay guidebooks almost always alert their readers to the ripeness of possibility: "Mexicans are usually friendly, elegant, and very dignified," says the 1990–91 edition of *Spartacus*. "Don't be surprised to be greeted with meaningful glances from the passing men.") The gay/lesbian political movement in Mexico started almost a decade later than its counterpart in the United States and has not yet become very large. The number of gay institutions (bars and other businesses, periodicals, organizations) remains relatively small, their life expectancy short.

On the other hand, there are no laws against homosexuality. Police in the cities have to invoke regulations about creating a disturbance or "public immorality" when they want to shake down the clients of a bar or stage a *redada* (raid) at a public bathhouse. Until *very* recently, there were not many bashings or murders where the motive appeared to be homophobia.

And despite the lack of formal organizations or a mass political social movement, Mexico has maintained a modest sort of homosexual *tradition*. Poets who write erotic lyrics to people of their own sex receive national prizes and kisses on the cheek from presidents of the Republic, acts duly noted by those who refer to themselves as being *de ambiente* or "in the life." They also say they are *de onda* (literally "of the wave," figuratively "in the scene"). As a term for their milieu, *puteria* (sexual looseness, sleaziness) may seem loaded with self-loathing, but among male homosexuals the usage can be fond, campy. And just as there are demeaning terms for *pasivos* in the straight world, in ambiente there are also sarcastic names for the *activo*. He is a *mayate*, "trade," or a *buga*, a "straight guy" (not from the English word *bugger*, as some gringos suppose, but more likely from *burgesa* [townsman or bourgeois]; there is a bar in Mexico City called Bugalandia). If a man "works both sides of the street," and especially if he hustles women as well as men, in many locales he is a *chichifo*.

Some of Joe Carrier's original informants insisted that for them the active/passive distinction was absolute. Others would take both roles, but had a distinct preference for being "top" or "bottom," depending on the *kind* of man they were with. Someone who had sex both ways or engaged in oral as well as anal sex was called an *internacional*, both because of his split allegiances and because he must have learned his exotic behavior somewhere outside Mexico. Folk wisdom on the subject includes a rich, circuitous understanding that we don't know what our desires are until we've tried them out. Clark Taylor, the second anthropologist to write on Mexican homosexual life, quotes a hard-to-translate saying: "*En gustos se rompen géneros, y en el petate culos*" (In pleasures genders break down, and on the mat assholes; or, Pleasure busts stereotypes, and bed butts). A *quimera* (chimera) is someone who doesn't know whether he likes women or men. Another name for an *internacional* is a *disco*, so called because he flips roles like a phonograph record. A man who changes his preference, moving from *activo* to *pasivo*, becomes an *hechizo* (a make-over).

The notion that for men the movement from active to passive is a one-way street is only speculative. What is more clear from the way SIDA is spreading in Mexico is that there must be many men who are "penetrators" when they are having vaginal or anal sex with their wives and who like to be the *pasivo* when having anal intercourse with another man. When I mentioned to Joe Carrier that it seems the active/passive division did not seem very rigid in Yucatán, he said, "Well, I've always thought that there would be differences, particularly in the south, where there's less emphasis on Spanish-style *machismo* and where the influence of the Indian cultures remains a lot stronger."

The man's nickname was "Pachi," his wife's name I didn't catch. I was introduced to them two years ago in 1990 at a workshop for people with VIH disease. The meeting took place on a Saturday afternoon around an oilcloth-covered table in the high-ceilinged old house that serves as headquarters for the Asociación Ya'ax Che, Mérida's tiny volunteer SIDA organization.

Both of them were fresh from bathing, their hair combed wet. Pachi was thickset and big, wearing an open-neck, big-print Hawaiian shirt and the gold chains and medallions traditional for Yucatec men. His wife had on a brown print dress with a little white collar. She had brown curly hair and was plump. I learned that Pachi worked as a driver, delivering beer for one of the big distributors. But who was seropositive? Both of them? There were no signs, except perhaps the thinness—more the tautness of the skin—around the man's jaw.

Alejandro Guerrero was president of the organization at the time, and he ran the meeting. A man named Ramiro Terrones, who has since died, was getting ready to go off to Mexico City to a training conference sponsored jointly by the Mexican federal agency CONASIDA and the University of California at San Francisco. Pachi asked politely how far Ramiro was planning to travel this evening. To Villahermosa? Oh no, Ramiro said, he'd be flying.

Oh. Some laughter around the table at the truck driver's expense. Pachi smiled, joined in a little.

Alejandro was to the big man's right. In a lull in the other conversation, Pachi began a low-voiced report to the doctor on how he was doing. He was well, he said, except for this eye business. He didn't rub his eye, but his fingers kept moving up to it, and he put his head back several times as though the eye had something in it. I couldn't see anything wrong, except perhaps that Pachi's eye was a little bloodshot. When he mentioned that his weight was up, Alejandro told him he should be glad of that.

"I am, Doctor, I am," he said.

A few minutes later, Pachi told me he was afraid of losing his job. At the place he worked, if they found out (he corrected himself, "*when* they find out—") he'd be fired for sure. Or if not fired, at least the other workers would keep their distance from him. "Since I've been sick," he said, "I've tried a number of times to let some of my friends know. When it comes up, I say, 'Well, what if *I* were to have it?' and they all just make fun of me, or even begin to avoid me, not have as much to do with me, just because I mention the subject.

"There is one guy I work with," he went on, "who's got a really messed-up sex life" (*una vida sexual muy desorganizada* was his phrase). "And sometimes I start to wonder if maybe *he* doesn't have it too. It's quite possible he does, and he just goes right on having sex without any kind of protection. Because you know, in the kind of work I do the guys are out traveling all the time and they pick girls up along the road and give them a ride, and *desgraciadamente* (unfortunately) for that they expect favors."

Pachi's wife turned to me. "Part of the problem is that everyone here in Yucatán gossips all the time," she said. "They just pass the news along about anything. Whether it's true or not, they don't care."

"Very different than in the United States with all its laws to protect the individual's privacy," Alejandro said. Some of his medical colleagues couldn't see why you couldn't just *take* a test on anyone you were suspicious of being seropositive, whether the patient wanted it or not.

Pachi was listening attentively. "Are these *seropositivos* also people who have the virus?" he asked.

"Well, the antibodies at least," Alejandro said.

"And me, Doctor? Am I seropositive?"

"Yes, Pachi, you are."

"And does everyone who has the virus in them necessarily advance to SIDA?"

That hadn't been completely proven yet, Alejandro said, but it seemed so, yes, in time.

A few minutes later, Pachi announced, "Well, Doctor, I think I'll be going." But he didn't go. A medical student came in to pick up materials to take to sex-education classes he was to give at a secondary school on Monday. Out of the corner of her eye, Pachi's wife watched the pamphlets being dealt out into piles and the condoms being put in smaller boxes.

Alejandro said to Pachi, "Are you still drinking your beer?"

"Oh yes," Pachi and his wife both nodded. She repeated, "I'm feeding him his beer." Then she reddened and looked down, as though the attention she had brought to herself was too much.

Finally, they stood up and we all stood and everyone around the table shook hands. Pachi asked would there be a meeting next Saturday. No, Alejandro said, because Ramiro would still be in Mexico City. And it seemed something else created a conflict the following week as well. So no meeting then either. Though Pachi and his wife took this news with good grace, they had trouble hiding their disappointment.

Soon after that, Alejandro and I had a talk about the problems involved in learning about people's sexual lives. He said, "Doctors certainly receive no training in how to do it."

He told me he had asked some of his women clients if they had ever had anal intercourse with their husbands. Some said their husbands may have proposed it once, but they had refused. Alejandro wondered if they always refuse.

I asked did he advise people who are positive for VIH to continue with their sex lives. People like the couple I met the other day, Pachi and his wife? "Yes," Alejandro said. "They have sex about once a week now, they say, or every other week. The wife was the one who originally tested positive. She rejected her husband, but then her result was found to be false. When they first appeared at my office, her brother was with them. He had come along to denounce Pachi's sins, all of them, which it seems Pachi had confessed—that he is an alcoholic, that he went to prostitutes, that he had sex with other men. I don't know, sometimes I think he may well continue these practices now."

"I was a surgical instruments specialist," José Manuel says. "That was what I was trained for, what I did. At the Juárez Hospital. And what happened was I went and took the test for VIH, and the people who administered it were friends of the women I worked with in surgery. So they told their friends and I came to work and my result was all over the place. Everyone else knew the news before I did. And they didn't want me around anymore. 'Get out of here,' they told me. I was devastated. I didn't know what to do. That was three years ago. Then Alejandro found me, and this work has brought me back to life."

"Your family?"

"My family has been wonderful to me. Very supportive, Carter. I'm very lucky."

Growing up, he tells me, he didn't know about being homosexual, because he liked his girlfriends and he liked his boyfriends. José Manuel was the sixth child and first son of a civil engineer who worked for the state in the construction of roads and a woman from Pichucalco in Chiapas. When José Manuel was sixteen a neighbor named Carlos, who was twenty-eight, said to him, "Do you like me?"

José Manuel said, "Why?"

"Because I like you," Carlos said, "and I think you're gay."

José Manuel said, "Well, I *do* like you."

So this Carlos started coming by to see him and courting him, bringing José Manuel flowers, coming to pick him up in the morning to drive him to school. "Just the way a boy courts a girl," José Manuel says. And though they got a look at each other in the shower, because Carlos was on one soccer team and José Manuel on another, there wasn't any sex between them—until the night of José Manuel's seventeenth birthday.

After that, they were always together. When he was eighteen, José Manuel went to his father and said, "Look, I'm a homosexual and I'm going to move in with Carlos. I'm happy that way and I'm not going to change back. I'm not going to paint my eyelids or wear earrings or become a *travesti* (transvestite), so I won't disgrace you in that way." And his father accepted it. "This makes you happy, you know what you're doing," he said.

With José Manuel's mother, however, it was a different story. She said things like, "Now I won't have a son." But in just a little while she came around. She came and brought flowers to the house where José Manuel and Carlos were living.

Then, after they had been together eight years, Carlos told José Manuel he was going out with a girl. José Manuel didn't think much about it. Well, he figured, that's his right. Carlos had never kept *him* from going out; they had never put any prohibitions at all on each other. José Manuel told himself, "This will pass." But then Carlos came to him and said he wanted to get married to the girl he had been seeing.

"After that I didn't want to have anything more to do with him," José Manuel says.

"And now?"

"Now we're *compadres*. I baptized their little girl. I'm over there all the time. Carlos's wife knows everything about us, about me. When I found out I was VIH, I went and told them. And they've been a big help."

There is a client of the SIDA clinic at the T-1 who is a *comerciante* (traveling salesman). He and his girlfriend had gone off to Guatemala, or they were living in Guatemala, selling clothes. This was nine years ago, during the dictatorship of the Christian fundamentalist General Efraín Ríos Montt. They were stopped on the road by the police and made to show their papers, and then they were taken off to a camp near Guatemala City whose purpose seemed to be to train soldiers in terror and brutalization. They would bring in young military recruits and five or six of them at a time would force sex on the people imprisoned there, men and women both. The camp was run by a woman.

José Manuel doesn't believe this story. He says the client has told him several times that his preference is for men. But the client has also told Alejandro about the camp on three separate occasions and has shown him the sworn account (*denuncia*) he has made either to the police or the armed forces here in Mexico.

The poor man lives in Cancún now. Thirty-six years of age. Whether the woman is seropositive or not he doesn't know. They split up some time ago and he has lost touch with her.

Starting around noon, the restaurant across from the T-1 serves a *comida* consisting of a pasta or rice dish and a main course with meat or fish for about three dollars. José Manuel waits until he gets off at three o'clock and eats at home, and Russell often goes to his mother's for *comida*, but Alejandro has his here almost every day in the one room that is closed off and air conditioned.

Over coffee, I start recalling what I was taught thirty years ago about interviewing in anthropological fieldwork, how the style is necessarily different from social psychology and sociology where the questionnaire or interview schedule hold sway. In ethnography you don't usually want to trap people, prove that your "informants" are lying by unmasking their internal inconsistencies or their disagreements with one another. Because you are new, because you are ignorant (like a very small child of the culture, some say), you more or less have to take it on faith that everything a person chooses to tell you is true on some level. In the moment, it's more important to have people's trust—or at least for them to know that to some extent you understand what they are saying—than to get precise "answers" to your questions. If something is being withheld from you, there may be a good reason for that. Everything in time, you tell yourself, important not to *stress* the person you're talking with. The contradictions that arise are food for later discussion. More or less, I'd imagine, the same way a good physician conducts the interview with a patient.

"Not always," Alejandro says. "That man Roberto you met over at the ISSSTE hospital? It was his wife who got him here from Chetumal. Later, when I asked him where he thinks he contracted the disease, he said he was sure it was from a needle stick from a patient three or four years ago. I asked Roberto if he had ever had sexual relations with other men and he denied it. At the time he was very sick, so I didn't say anything more.

"Then the other day some other people came up from Chetumal to visit him, and one of them told me when Roberto first became a nurse he lived with one of the other male nurses for a year. When he was just seventeen or so. It made me wonder if he hadn't had a sexual relationship then that he doesn't want to talk about now. So I told him, 'Roberto, you know, this thing about the needle stick is very important. If that *is* how you got infected, you'll be one of the very few cases in Mexico—in the world, actually—and the nurses in all the hospitals will hear about your case and they'll be afraid of dealing with patients who have SIDA.' "

"What did Roberto say?"

"Nothing. He just got very nervous and began to sweat, and then he began to cry."

"Maybe he'll say something to you later."

"Maybe he will," Alejandro says.

To know you are HIV-positive is to have a secret. Over time (a short time, a long time) your secret is almost bound to get out. And though in the beginning your new knowledge may not seem like knowledge at all but chaos, in time you begin to gain some control over it. You begin to figure out who you want to tell, to be able to calculate some of the risks. The secret becomes a "fact," and you begin to manage it.

I know all this, I tell Alejandro, from watching my lover deal with the world over the last four years. And because, in a much lesser way, his secret has been my secret too.

Alejandro recalls a man who he thinks "simply shut his mouth." A young father. Alejandro is convinced the man took the VIH test back in November and just didn't tell anyone the result. Now it is the next to last week of March. Three days ago the man showed up at the hospital very ill, confused. Neurological impairments. Yesterday he died. Alejandro spoke with the wife. She said most of her husband's friends were homosexuals, maybe that was how he got the disease.

"At the present moment," Alejandro says, "even without a cure, or even really long-lasting forms of treatment, that man's way of dealing with it was clearly a form of suicide."

While I am familiar with some of the symptoms Alejandro's and Russell's patients present with (pneumocystis pneumonia, chronic diarrhea, chronically infected lymph glands), others reflect not only the tropical climate but a very different way of living. Rapid weight loss, which they call here *desgaste* (wasting disease), can advance much farther than it might in the States without being noticed. Many people in the Yucatán are malnourished or suffer from other diseases that may also cause wasting. Alejandro has had patients who lost half their body weight before anyone thought to bring them to a clinic. Tuberculosis—in other parts of the body as well as the lungs—is a big problem. Alejandro speaks also of *astenia* (asthenia or general debility).

Before Alejandro and Russell began administering the antiviral retrovir (AZT) at the T-1, patients complained of peripheral neuropathy—aching limbs, hands, and feet. When they hurt now, especially in their leg muscles, it is probably the effect of the drug itself. "It's a trade-off," Alejandro says. The treatment for peripheral neuropathy they use is the vitamin *Pyridoxina*, which is also put in combination with anti-TB drugs.

For pneumocystis pneumonia, they treat with the antibiotic Bactrin. Alejandro knows about the struggles with the insurance companies to get aerosolized pentamidine admitted as a legitimate treatment in the States several years ago, but the matter doesn't concern him much because there is not much pentamidine available in Mexico to administer in any form. Gancylovir, which is usually effective against outbreaks of herpes zoster, is also very hard to get.

Alejandro has had AZT for almost two years. In that time he and Russell have used it with eighty-six clients, sixty-five of whom are still living. Some are also taking acyclovir, which is thought to have a positive synergistic effect when used in combination with AZT. Alpha interferon A is given intramuscularly to some clients (the brand name of the product is *Intrón A*). The syringes and needles are often handed over to clients so the medication can be administered by someone at home or by a neighbor: illegal injection drug use remains such a small problem in Mexico that there are no laws against having "works" in your possession. Until the spring of 1992, Alejandro and Russell had no access to either ddI (dideoxyinosine) or ddC (dideoxycytidine). The small amounts of ddI they have now were donated by doctors in the States. Still no ddC.

The cost of a frasco of AZT (a hundred capsules), which Burroughs-Wellcome de Mexico sells to IMSS at wholesale, is 380,000 pesos or about U.S. $125. (The commercial price in Mexico is 580,000 pesos or U.S. $186.) Alejandro's records show that in less than two years his clinic has handed out 836 frascos. In dollars, this means the medication has cost U.S. $104,500. (He has also been giving it to his patients at the ISSSTE hospital, so the grand total is actually a good deal higher.) Though he does nothing to hide the facts, Alejandro wonders when the amounts they have been spending will be noticed by IMSS central accounting, and what the response will be, especially if the matter gets into the press.

Recently, he has been pulling together a large set of graphs that demonstrate how AZT has extended their patients' lives. The first people who appeared at the T-1 with symptoms of SIDA all died within a year. Now, with earlier diagnosis, AZT, and new treatments for the opportunistic infections, life expectancy for men with the disease has risen to more than two-and-a-half years. Women tend to be diagnosed later in the course of the illness. Their life expectancy has gone up, too, but only to about a year. Alejandro is clearly betting on his figures to justify not only his pharmacy bill but his entire clinic.

One quirk in the eligibility law may make a difference. In order to become a *vigente* at IMSS, a person needs to be employed more than fifteen days in a business that contributes to the Social Security System. In 1982 a modification of the Social Security law provided for people with transmissible chronic illnesses, which would include TB and sexually transmitted diseases like syphilis—and SIDA—to be kept in the system indefinitely. "A real piece of luck," Alejandro says, especially since 1982 was the year *before* the first cases of SIDA were reported in Mexico.

As a student at the University of Yucatán Russell was heavily involved in theater and dance. Even today, going upstairs to do rounds, or even just on the way to meet his Wednesday morning clinic hours, which begin at eight, he likes to make a dramatic impression, sinking his hands deep in his coat pockets and taking big, hurried steps, his head down, his black eyes looking up from under darkened brows.

His patients are a mixed group, mostly people with VIH disease, but through the morning he also sees some other referrals. His nurse, Magdalena Estrellas, is a bustly little person in her forties with some blond-red in her hair. The examining room is small and filled with furniture, a desk for the doctor, a chair for the patient, two extra chairs, an examining table, a glass-front metal bookcase piled high with files and papers.

Russell sits with one leg tucked under himself, or both feet bouncing nervously on the floor under the desk. Hugo Vargas, a broad-faced, shy, twenty-nine-year-old health *promotor*, or outreach worker, is also in the room this morning, but Russell usually says nothing to his patients to explain either Hugo's or my presence here. When there is a pause, or when Russell goes out for a minute, I sometimes tell them my name, and that I'm a colleague of Alejandro and Russell from the States.

The first young man to come in is named Narciso. He is suffering from a skin disease, red blotches all over his chest and arms. He has been to Mexico City recently to take the T helper cell test again. He announces he has only six T cells left. Down from sixty eight months ago. He still goes to work, he says. Does he still drink? A little, he says. Sex? Well— Narciso says. Russell shrugs and says, "Have sex if you want, as long as it's safe, but you really shouldn't be drinking at all anymore, you know."

Next comes a willowy, alert, tan young man with a canvas bag over his shoulder and a soft white rayon shirt whom Russell does choose to introduce. Ramón. We get up, shake hands, sit back down. "Ramón here is one of the best dancers we have," Russell says. Ramón performs in the "folklorico" at one of the hotels in Cancún. Worked last night—there is only one show each evening—then took the bus across the peninsula. What time did you leave there? I ask. He took the 12:30, Ramón says. Which means he got here around 5:00 A.M.

"Are you eating, Ramón?" Russell asks.

"Yes."

"How? Give me an example. What did you eat yesterday?"

Ramón has to think a minute. "At breakfast, some cereal with fruit, then in the afternoon a piece of meat—a beefsteak—with vegetables and rice. Something before the show, a snack, not much."

"And since then?"

"Nothing much, a Coke, a sandwich at the bus depot in Cancún."

He sweats in the night, he says, and his muscles ache after his performances, but he can still keep up. Russell says, "You're not going to be able to go on dancing forever, Ramón. You know that, don't you?"

"Yes, I do. But for the time being—"

His voice trails off. Russell looks down at Ramón's file.

"Come, let's examine you."

Ramón takes off his shirt and Russell listens to his chest with a stethoscope. Ramón then gets on the examining table and lets his pants down to his knees. He is wearing blue bikini undershorts. Russell feels all around his abdomen, down to the edge of his pubic hair. When he's dressed again and ready to go, Russell says, "Come back, Ramón."

"I will, Doctor."

With every client, Russell has paperwork. Little notations in the file, often a slip of paper patients bring with them that needs to be written on or signed or separated from its carbons, then at the end of the visit almost always at least one prescription and an order to fill out. The prescription books are numbered, and sometimes Russell can't find one. There are stamps too. He writes vigorously, then stamps vigorously, in a hurry, bang bang bang!! THERE! Rips off the copy for the client and hands it over with a flourish.

Another young man arrives—twenty-three or twenty-four—with a cough. He has bad tonsils, he says. Russell takes a tongue depressor and checks them, writes a prescription, tells him to come back in a week.

Next is a married couple, probably in their thirties. He is tall, has on a nicely pressed and starched white shirt, slacks. Her densely curled hair is glossy with gel. Short check skirt, halter top, made up with mascara and pencil so she looks continually surprised. They sit holding hands. He is the one who is VIH-positive. At first the visit seems to be a general health checkup, and the wife does most of the talking. But then suddenly the man says he's been getting pains down in the area of his liver. Russell has him get up on the examining table and undo his pants, then presses all over his abdomen. When he's done, the man gets up and sits again.

Russell asks this man, too, to tell him what he eats in a day. "Just generally speaking," Russell adds.

The man has to think. He mentions eggs and toast and juice in the morning when he's home, with a glass of milk to drink. Meat at midday—

"With bread?" Russell asks.

"Yes. Some kind of roll, usually." Then at night, he says, just coffee with milk and a sweet roll or, if he and his wife go out, some pizza or maybe a hamburger. "I'm trying to eat more fruits and vegetables," he says, "but I travel for my company, in my own car, and it's hard, you know. I have to stop and eat in some town or another, and meat and bread are really all there is. It's after I've been driving around sometimes that I get the pain in my side."

Russell fixes an eye on both of them, pauses. The husband is eating too much meat, he says. Needs more vegetables and fruit. He should try peanuts when he's hungry, without too much salt they're full of protein and good for you. "Also, you're eating too much bread made from wheat. In a situation like yours, it can block up your stomach. Try to stay away from so much of it."

Then abruptly he asks is their sex life all right. Husband and wife look at each other, laugh. Yes, they say, fine. "Although—" The man's been wondering. It seems that since he got this disease there's more fluid coming out of him in the early part of lovemaking. Is there anything wrong with that?

Russell says, "Don't worry about it."

He takes his time with these people. They're supposed to go to the D.F. soon for the husband to have a new T cell test, but there's been a problem about that at his job. He sells medical supplies, and when his supervisor came from Mexico City he noticed on something—a work excuse—that Russell's stamp said *INFECTOLOGÍA*. The supervisor asked him what he had to go to Mexico City for. "What can I tell him, Doctor?"

Russell thinks for a minute. "Tell him you have to be tested for hepatitis. That will do."

José Manuel's rap about nutrition is similar to Russell's. You have to start thinking about what you eat all the time, he tells his VIH-positive people, make sure you get the things your body needs. More protein, from eggs, from fish. Generally, you won't need as much starch—bread and wheat products—as you used to. José Manuel recommends *jalea real* (queen bee jelly) to everyone. "Available right here in health food stores and a natural product of our own Yucatán," he says, putting on the glassy voice of a television huckster. "Some people mix it up in something, but I just eat it right out of the jar in the morning with a spoon!"

Hugo Vargas is big for a Yucatec, five feet nine or ten. Mustache, thick neck. For exercise he lifts weights, he tells us. He has begun coming around because his previous work has ended, and he wonders if there isn't a chance they could take him on at the SIDA clinic here. He was trained in emergency medicine, and his last job was as a *promotor* in the recent cholera outbreak. They covered villages throughout Yucatán and down into Campeche. In cholera, Hugo says, you vomit over and over and your shit turns white and runny. Then you have to get to a hospital quickly. The main danger is dehydration, then complications. Old people and children are at the most risk. In addition to a little English, Hugo knows a few expressions in Maya. "*Tu'ux cabin?*" (Where are you going?) he says, deepening his voice. And "*Co'oten hanal!*" (Come to eat). Alejandro, Russell, and José Manuel send him on errands. He trots off to deliver the VIH-test blood to the laboratory, across the street to get Cokes. Each morning he shows up in a fresh, beautifully ironed white shirt. He lives with his mother on the north side of the city. Although he has only been around a few days, José Manuel has been working assiduously on the question of Hugo's sexual preferences. His conclusion is "*Ni picha, ni cacha, ni deja a batear*" (Doesn't pitch, doesn't catch, doesn't come up to bat). Head down, deferential, Hugo follows along when Russell goes up to the third floor before noon to make his rounds. A guard is posted at the glass doors before you get to the elevators. A civilian blocks the path, arguing with the guard. We have to go around them.

"Standing in the way. It's a Mexican national habit," Russell says.

"They do it in my country too," I tell him.

The three current SIDA inpatients at the T-1 are all together in the same four-bed room. Although the nurses wear rubber gloves when they are cleaning people up or changing sheets, no isolation precautions are taken. (When I ask Alejandro what the difference is, he says only that the ISSSTE hospital hasn't had people with SIDA as long as the T-1.) Lunch, served on covered plastic plates, has already come up. Apples, soup, Jello, bread, spaghetti, the amounts smaller than at a U.S. hospital.

First inside the door is Miguel. He has been here nearly a month this time. Pneumocystis and probably TB. He is on oxygen, hard to understand with the plastic mask over his nose and mouth. Sweaty much of the time, his hair wet, plastered back. His mother is usually present to tend him, make his wants known to the doctor. Miguel has a portable television playing constantly on his bed table and an electric fan blowing on him. The chili and other foods his mother brings from home are in plastic containers. There is a folding aluminum chair for her to sit on against the wall. In her big distressed eyes, the mother looks like her son.

Next to Miguel is Jorge Dario Valle, a man in his thirties. He is on an IV drip. Passed out, thin, barely covered by his sheet. Wearing socks. Jorge Dario has a boxer's face, a wide nose and thick lips, receding reddish hair, a stubble beard. The nurses say they can't wake him. Jorge's mother is present, a little woman in a mestiza's *huipil*, light-skinned like her son, tight gray curls all over her head. "He was awake in the night," she tells the doctor. "He *couldn't* sleep then."

Russell calls his name aloud. "JORGE DARIO VALLE! JORGE?! Are you here or not?" Russell comes closer, squeezes Jorge's left leg, then the right. Jorge has advanced syphilis. He is paralyzed down his entire left side. "Look at this," Russell tells Hugo Vargas, pulling up an eyelid, letting it go. "This is not involuntary, it's willful. Valle? Are you in there, man?"

Nothing. The eye Russell has revealed is gray-green, lustrous but still.

Closest to the window is Juanito, thirty-one or thirty-two. The view is out across the low houses, the trees, east to the green plain. Juanito is very thin, long-haired, tall (or so it seems from his length in the bed, since I haven't seen him standing up). Big eyes, high forehead. His mother is here also, a woman in her late forties or early fifties with long, bushy gray hair.

Juanito has a huge swelling on the lower left side of his abdomen. Over the weekend they began draining it. By Monday they had gotten six liters of a brownish fluid out of him. The bottles on the floor under the bed are filled to the top. Russell holds one up to the light, turns it, showing the liquid to me. It is viscous, opaque, the color of tamarind. "See all the yellow in it?" he says. Russell has been having trouble getting anyone to analyze this stuff. He palpates Juanito's abdomen, but nothing seems to hurt especially. This patient is also wearing skimpy blue bikini shorts, and the skin of his belly is bright pink from being so distended.

"I'm going to keep you another ten days," says Russell.

Juanito says, "Why are you doing that to me? What is there in this place for me?"

Russell doesn't answer him.

Then Juanito complains of being nervous and upset. His hands move lightly along his body as he talks.

"I'll send someone up to see you," Russell promises, already in motion toward the door.

Once he has been through the ward, Russell takes the patients' charts, which are kept in spring-top clutch metal holders, into a small room with two desks, two manual typewriters, a computer terminal, telephones, an ashtray. On a shelf are copies of diagnostic manuals in English and Spanish, medical journals. On the wall two posters: a Winston Churchill quote, "One of the tragedies of our century is that instead of being USEFUL, people want to be IMPORTANT"; the other Lucy giving Charlie Brown a kiss and the motto, "Every now and then, EVERYBODY needs a stimulant." Russell takes one of the machines, runs a patient's current order in, types madly with both index fingers. Other doctors stand around, some of them younger, offering opinions to one another, talking on the phone. Russell asks for advice on one case. I am introduced to Hugo Cabrera, the doctor who saw the first two cases of SIDA in Yucatán back in 1983, a big, dark-haired man. Several of the doctors smoke. Russell bums a cigarette while he types.

His daily orders are full of medications. The SIDA patients all seem to be on eight or nine different drugs at all times. At other hours of the day the orders are written up by residents, who seem generally to continue whatever the doctor has prescribed before. Often the entry ends with the word *grave* (serious).

Juanito is a special worry to them. Alejandro refers to Juanito's TB, but Russell sets that idea aside and continues to speak about the problem of the peritonitis. "The gastrointestinal track has just shut down," Russell tells me. He is frustrated. "I have asked three different surgeons to operate on this boy, including my *cuates* (pals), and none of them is willing to do it. So what can *I* do? Send him home to die. That's it."

We are back downstairs. Suddenly Russell motions to me and we start off at a clip toward a set of consulting rooms at the other end of the hall. "Now, Charlie, we're going to the psychiatrist," Russell laughs. "But don't worry, it's not for treatment."

He knocks repeatedly, but "David," the psychiatrist he hoped he could get to deal with Juanito's nervousness, isn't there. So before he goes off for the day himself, Russell returns to the office and asks José Manuel if *he'll* make a trip upstairs to see what *he* can do.

At the end of his shift, José Manuel and I take the elevator back up to the third floor. "It's a shame seeing Juanito the way he is today," he tells me. "He was *so* beautiful before. He had this fine, fine skin he treated with creams and black, black hair, and when he dressed up he always had all the best-looking clothes. He would be invited into girls' sewing classes, Carter, to show off the latest styles. He knew all about those things, and how to do them. He was a singer, a *travesti*, in only the best shows."

But once out into the yellow tile hall, José Manuel becomes all efficiency again. He *breezes* into the room. "What's this I hear, Juanito? You're unhappy? Don't you have everything you could ever need here?"

Juanito looks around, spreading his long hands to take in the whole scene, smiles ironically toward José Manuel.

"Then where do you think you're going so fast?" José Manuel asks. "If you have a date waiting for you, just tell me, OK? We should start getting you ready."

Later, in the evening, Alejandro is hopeful about the situation. He has talked to other members of the surgical staff and maybe one of them will operate on Juanito. We are having a nine o'clock supper at the POP, a coffee shop and restaurant downtown across from the university. I eat a sandwich of steak strips with peppers and cheese, and Alejandro is dipping pieces of french bread into a bubbly cheese fondue. He says, "I think of Juanito as someone who carries his 'self' in a small vessel, bearing it before him. And I keep wondering how I'm going to tell him that a mountain of rocks is going to come down on his head. But you know, I don't think it matters. I don't think Juanito's going to lose that precious vessel of himself no matter what happens."

Some doctors I know at home act as though to set foot outside the boundaries of the United States is to put your life in desperate peril. For even a ten-day trip abroad, they protect themselves by going on a major course of antibiotics as prophylaxis. The incompetent Third-

World doctor, especially the Mexican one, alcoholic, misogynistic, sadistic or at the least devil-may-care or just plain ignorant, is a recurrent bogeyman of gringo travel lore. Whatever criticism we may have of our own medical care system, we have bought—without question—the idea that it is not only the best, it is the *only* care that will do for us.

Columnist Alexander Cockburn has a funny bit where he notes how often he sees a newspaper filler he calls "Fifty-five in Delhi Bus." Never longer than a paragraph or two, the piece records a staggering loss of life from a bus in India going into the river, off the road, over the edge. Some day, Cockburn says, he wants to follow up on one of these stories. Is it true? Do busses crash with such enormous regularity in India? And why is there never any *deeper* explanation of what has happened? No mention of something like the World Bank consistently refusing India loans to improve its roads because of the country's bad credit rating, or defective used busses from the West being sold off to the unsuspecting nations.

Whether or not the Delhi bus tragedy ever actually takes place, Cockburn thinks the *reason* the filler appears with such regularity in our papers is to remind us that, whatever the liabilities, we do live in a "first" world where these appalling disasters don't occur, or at least not so frequently.

My Sicilian-American friend Cosimo Corsano was talking about quitting his job early and retiring to Puerto Rico. Why didn't I do the same, he asked. I would like to, I said, but living with someone who was HIV-positive I didn't think it was possible for us. Travel has always made Ray anxious, and now he doesn't want to go places where the risk of getting sick is so much higher.

"But Carter," Cosimo said, "we are all going to rot away. Why not in a pleasant setting, one where they are kind to old men?"

It seems to me that on balance the care for VIH-positive clients at the Hospital T-1 in Mérida is good when compared to what many HIV clients receive in some of the larger cities of California. It is much easier to get in to see Russell Rodriguez or Alejandro Guerrero at IMSS than it is to get an appointment with an AIDS doctor at many of the swamped public clinics of San Francisco, New York, or Los Angeles. (At one point the wait at the Los Angeles County Public Health clinic devoted to AIDS was said to be, on average, five hours.) For patients who have to be hospitalized at the T-1, plenty of adequate medication is available. The nursing care seems at least as efficient and humane as what you would get in a U.S. hospital. The atmosphere on the third floor is good, family and close friends have plenty of access to the patients. Without as much technology at hand, Alejandro and Russell are able to order fewer of the major diagnostic procedures than their North American counterparts would (for example, CAT scans are available, but the hospital is not equipped with the multimillion dollar machinery needed for Magnetic Resonance Imaging). They do less blood work on patients at the T-1 than might be done in the United States. Most of the same tests are available, but they are run less frequently. Certainly, having to go all the way to Mexico City for a T helper cell test wastes both funds and the patients' precious cache of health. Alejandro and Russell are frustrated by the fact that they haven't been able to convince the hospital's pathologists to perform autopsies on some of their more baffling cases. If they could, they might be able to treat others more intelligently in the future.

IMSS has a system called ADEC (Atención Domiciliaria Enfermos Crónicos), which sends nurses three days a week to see people at home who are paralyzed (hemiplegics) or who have cancer. Although José Manuel often takes it on himself to go provide critical services to regulars from his clinic in their final days, ADEC generally has not been much help to SIDA patients, who are likely to need some attention every twenty-four hours.

Very little formal psychological assistance is being offered to people who are VIH-positive, or to the families, lovers, and friends affected by their illness or their death. The private Asociación Ya'ax Che sponsors *grupos de autoapoyo* (self-help groups), but they have had trouble getting professional psychologists to volunteer to lead them. Nationally, a movement is starting in which people with VIH disease are fighting against the loss of civil rights because of their illness, but the positive effects of this struggle have not yet been felt in Yucatán.

Alejandro is proud of what he has been able to accomplish. (When I asked him what *he* would call a piece about his clinic, he said promptly, "*Los adelantados*," which can translate as "those out in front" or "the forerunners.") His operation at the T-1 disturbs the status quo because it links a fairly well-funded and visible medical and public health effort to the cause of people who are stigmatized (not just homosexuals, but anyone with SIDA). The clinic's very existence creates discomfort among straight people—other doctors, administrators, some clients. Some members of the public complain about Alejandro's and Russell's patients because of their flamboyance in the waiting rooms, their wild clothes, even their excessive use of scent. In the beginning some nurses and staff had fears about dealing with people with SIDA, but unlike the physicians, they lack the resources—the privilege—to wash their hands of these patients.

José Manuel has friends, a little redhead named Niko and her partner Stella. Both work at the T-1, Stella in administration and Niko as a nurse, usually assigned to the third floor. José Manuel's friendship with Niko goes back at least as far as the years they were both at the Juárez Hospital, before José Manuel was thrown out of there for being VIH-positive. In those days, he and Niko were a kind of couple, always going out drinking and dancing together with their straight friends from work. Niko was married once and has a little boy, eight or nine. She showed me the little photo of him she keeps in a translucent plastic heart on her key ring. Stella, a smoky, tall blond with long hair in ringlets, is only the second woman Niko has gone with.

I ask them why the doctors sometimes reject the SIDA patients but the nurses and technical staff don't. Neither of them has a solid answer to the question, but it is clear to me that they watch the treatment of gay men at the T-1 with great care. "It is disrespectful what some of those doctors will try to get away with," Niko says, "when they think no one who cares is looking—" Niko and Stella both tune in on my question because they are aware at some level that it applies to them too, gives them an indication of how they are valued in the world where they work.

Alejandro has the expertise and the politics—including his open, unjudging stances concerning many aspects of sexuality—to make him an effective head of his hospital's "Activities Against SIDA." From what I can tell, the other doctors fully respect him for his knowledge of infectious disease. Besides his professional credentials, being raised in the milieu of the national military and governmental elite seems to give him a sense of independence when it is his job to set policy. Though he generally distrusts professional politicians, including those in the Mexican public health establishment, he recognizes that in his own way he also is "political."

His chief liability seems to be that, in spite of all the years he has lived in the Yucatán, he is not a member of the provincial oligarchy from which leaders in every field, including medicine, come. The ruling class's resistance to the peninsula's absorption into the nation has a long history. "*Our* Yucatán" they still call it, meaning two things: not just one of the states of the Republic, but actually a country by itself, the old, idealized, vastly pleasant and trouble-free "land of the pheasant and the deer," as Bishop Landa's *Relación* says the Maya called it; and also "theirs" in the sense of being a place entirely owned and governed by themselves and not subject to the intrusions of any outsiders, either from Mexico City or from abroad.

On the social level, Alejandro has taken none of the steps that might cause the establishment doctors to bring him into their circle. He does not belong to a country club or go sports shooting or fishing on the weekend. He is still at enough distance to be able to hear the peculiar, older ways they use certain Spanish verbs here: *Prestar*, for example, means not only "to lend," but also "to borrow." *Buscar* is "to look for" and also "to find," which means a Yucatec would be perfectly capable of saying the apparently nonsensical sentence, "*Te buscaba, pero ya te busque*" (I was looking for you, but now I've found you).

There is a woman, twenty-four, named Lupita. Her husband was the one who infected her, and he has died. She got a new lover and told him she had SIDA, but she is a big-breasted, fleshy woman and the man wouldn't believe her and wouldn't wear a condom. She got pregnant and came to Alejandro. He put the problem to the obstetrics and gynecology staff, many of whom are strong Catholics and *Pro Vida* (Pro Life). They held a big meeting where Alejandro was the only one present in favor of Lupita getting an abortion. "She knew she had SIDA," the others said. "This is her responsibility, not ours." So Lupita went to a *rinconera* (neighborhood abortionist), and the business was botched. She showed up at the hospital bleeding. So the same doctors who had refused to perform what is called a *legrado* the first time now had to do it at much greater risk to the patient (and to themselves). And because the patient said she wanted it, the doctors now decided they would also perform a tubal ligature.

But then Lupita showed up at Alejandro's office pregnant again. How did this happen? Oh, the other doctors said, they *forgot* the tubal ligature or for some reason they *couldn't* do it, or—whatever.

A private professional abortion costs between a million and 1.5 million pesos (U.S. $330–$495). Working in a shop, a woman Lupita's age might earn U.S. $.60 an hour, or $5.00 or $6.00 a day.

Alejandro goes up into the administrative offices to give a talk on SIDA in the workplace. The audience in the small classroom is twenty-five or so men and women, including nurses, secretaries, people from the kitchen and maintenance. Alejandro wants to use the blackboard, but there is no chalk. Sessions are going on in several rooms around us, and while the organizer of this one is out trying to borrow a piece of chalk, somebody else darts in and bears off the only eraser on the sill. Everyone is still laughing about that when the organizer returns triumphant with a tiny stub of chalk.

"In any business or organization," Alejandro begins, "in exchange for your labor what you get is a salary, obviously. But you should also get some—" and he writes it up—"SECURITY. For what you give of your time and effort, you should be able to *demand* certain things in exchange. But in order to get what you deserve in terms of security and safe conditions on the job, *you* have to have some knowledge of what it is you need, and that demands having some education.

"Working in a hospital we encounter certain problems concerning our personal health and safety that you don't always find in other locations. What are they? Well, funguses, viruses, and bacteria are the three we have to worry about. What are the ways they enter the body? Through the skin (as cuts), by breathing them (the streptococci, the staphylococci, tuberculosis), and through blood, the mucosa, the digestive tract. It's not pleasant to think about," he says, "but when we get a bacterial infection it is often because we have eaten a very tiny piece of someone else's feces.

"In the area of infections we may get from our patients' blood, hepatitis is the one we usually think of," he reminds them, "although cirrhosis is also highly contagious. There are three kinds of hepatitis—A, which is not so serious, and B and C, which are. The point here is that hepatitis is a known infection, a risk we take, which we also know how to protect against. As is VIH. There are probably three million cases of SIDA in the world today. So far, in more than ten years, there have only been three hundred health workers who have been infected by it through their employment. None of these has been in Mexico. Still, since it is a fatal and awful disease, it is necessary for us to learn as much as we can about how to avoid it on the job."

Alejandro writes on the board—*PINCHAZOS*.

"Now some people think when they're handling a needle that has been in a patient with SIDA, the safest thing is to put the plastic cap back on after they've used it. But that's *not* a good idea, because of the great possibility that your attention will be drawn by something else while you're doing it and you'll end up sticking yourself for sure." Alejandro pantomimes becoming distracted and poking a needle into his own finger. "Simpler and safer just to throw the syringe and the cap out separately. Other needle sticks come about when maintenance workers lift trash bags that have needles in them, or when somebody lets a needle dangle and it punctures them either in their own or someone else's leg.

"If you get a needle stick," he advises, "you should take a VIH test immediately. If you are negative at first and then at six weeks you take another test and show up positive, you'll have as good a proof as we know that your illness was work-related. I recommend *four* tests, for hepatitis as well as VIH: in the first week, at six weeks, at three months, and at six months. Sometimes people who work here and who've been exposed come to ask us about the test, but then don't come back to take it. Why? I don't know. But I suspect it is sometimes out of fear that they may already be VIH-positive and still don't want to know.

"Why do we allow for confidentiality in this test? One time one of the nurses asked me, 'Why are you *protecting* these homosexuals?' I told her I wasn't only protecting homosexuals, I was protecting everyone who has a job—treating everyone else the way she would want to be treated, too."

Alejandro speaks about rejection of people with SIDA in the hospital. The times when kitchen workers didn't want to wash SIDA patients' dishes with other people's and how baseless that fear has turned out to be. He mentions people "rejected by the world, by their families, and even here, where they come to us looking for 'health,' also rejected."

Silence. Then the group begins asking Alejandro about education on SIDA. Why isn't the government doing more? Because, Alejandro responds, the government policy is—and he wipes the blackboard clear and writes the word *SILENCIO*. What about condoms? they ask. Don't some of the doctors say that condoms don't keep the virus out of our system? But these same doctors, Alejandro responds, like the rest of us, continue to wear rubber gloves to protect themselves when they are performing surgery. Why wear them at all if you don't believe rubber forms an effective barrier for diseases borne in blood?

Then why do the doctors spread such lies, the audience wants to know. Because, Alejandro says, the corollary of the policy of silence is—and he writes it up, off to the side—*DESINFORMACIÓN*.

He moves on to the four ways he knows of to avoid contracting SIDA through sex: abstention, reduction of the number of partners, the use of condoms, and avoidance of sex with people at greater risk—homosexuals and drug users. And there he ends.

Applause, thanks from the group, a few more questions, almost all of them from the nurses. On the way back downstairs, Alejandro says this is the usual case, the nurses are more forthright, aggressive, have more education than other staff people. I tell him I liked him taking it to the point he did, then letting them ask the protection and education questions about sex. "Yes," he says, "with this sort of group it usually works. And since I was asked to talk about risk in the workplace, this way no one can complain that I started talking about sex where I wasn't asked to."

He arrives around 9:30 one morning carrying a ledger, a young, blondish doctor, short hair, blue eyes, a plain white short-sleeve shirt and chinos, muscled arms, the physique of a gymnast or a runner. I am introduced to him but I don't remember his name. Everyone in the office knows him. I think he has worked with Alejandro and the others on a project. José Manuel is busy with something else, and apologizes. The young doctor sits easily at the round table in the center of the room. He can wait, he says. He joins us in a Coke, laughs about how warm it is and the rectangular hole in the wall where the air conditioner was. Alejandro says they've found a replacement, they're about to bring it over. "I used Carter," he claims, "told them I had visitors here from the United States and it was too hot for them to do their work."

José Manuel finishes what he has been doing finally and brings his own ledger from the files by his desk over to the round table. Both men open their books. The young doctor works for the government and has the job, among others, of keeping statistics on deaths from SIDA. His ledger has a set of columns across the page: name, age, sex, occupation, sexual preference, date of onset, progression to "Step IV," date and cause of death, others.

Many of the last names are Mayan. Or mixed, the father's surname Spanish, the mother's Mayan. Or the other way around. The doctor's records are by month, so he and José Manuel go back and forth, into last year, up to last week. Sometimes, probably because he already knows the cases, the doctor fills in some of his columns without even looking over onto José Manuel's ledger or asking.

Occupation? Housewife. Worker, guest house. Bartender. Police. Public accountant. Nurse.

José Manuel comments on the policeman. He lost a lot of weight and managed to keep it from the other people he was working with, almost to the end. A married man, but his wife isn't VIH, or his children.

Heterosexual. Homosexual. Bisexual.

"*Bisexual bicicleta*," says José Manuel.

Then, a minute later, about another entry, the doctor asks, "*Homosexual?*"

José Manuel nods, "*Homosexual promiscuo. Puerco. Puerco mañoso.*"

The young man José Manuel calls a conniving pig was a male nurse, and one of the people they weren't able to do much for. He arrived at the T-1 on a Friday and died the following Tuesday. He had lost a tremendous amount of weight, José Manuel says.

The statistician tells me in the state of Yucatán the number of dead is about 100, the number of those living with SIDA about 110, the number recognized as VIH-positive more or less 200.

He closes the ledger, sighs, gets up to go. A pleasant person. Everyone says, "Come again, *Doctor*, see you soon," and he takes his leave.

Then almost immediately the electrician appears, followed by the same six or seven maintenance men who removed the old air conditioner on Monday. They get up on the table and the filing cabinets and lift the replacement from their cart up into the hole in the wall and everyone claps. The others depart, and the electrician stays to hook up the new machine to the power box.

José Manuel tells me he went to the young male nurse's *velorio* (prayer service), and afterward the boy's father took him home with him. The place was full of different drugs. "Probably trying to medicate himself," José Manuel says. "What awful foolishness. Death to all homosexuals then!"

During the morning it clouds up and then rains, warm gushes of water, pattering, then thundering, then pattering again in the interior courtyards of the T-1.

A man and a woman come into Russell's office. The man is still heavy—heavier, actually—and handsome with his wide face, slicked-back hair, the almond eyes, broad mustache, formed mouth, thick, hairy forearms. Pachi's complexion is ruddy. His skin, though, is more papery than before, emphasizing the bones underneath. (An effect of taking the antivirals or of the disease itself? I still don't know.) Pachi's wife, too, has gained weight in the two years since I first met them at the Asociación Ya'ax Che. Her hair is still in curls and she looks a good deal older than I remember. Pachi has a little cough. He covers his mouth with his hand and turns away. Russell gets him up to weigh himself and they joke because the scale only goes to 100 kilos (220 pounds) and Pachi weighs more than that. He has come for a prescription he needs refilled. When the visit is over and they stand up to go, I stand too and say, "I think I know you."

Pachi nods, and his wife also brightens. "Yes, I thought it was you," he says.

"You were at a meeting I attended. Glad to see you again. And you're doing well?"

"I'm doing alright," Pachi shrugs.

"And you, señora?"

"Oh I'm fine," she says.

The next patient is a man they call Don Alberto, an affable fellow with big shoulders, big head, thinning hair, red sunburned skin, a mustache. He has on a boat-neck striped shirt and new stone-washed jeans. Prosperous-looking. Doing well, he says. Only problem today is tonsils.

Russell gets a tongue depressor. "Now open up, Don Alberto, and pretend this is something large and agreeable."

"Aaarg—ghh!" says Don Alberto as Russell holds his head back, moves the stick around. When it comes out, Don Alberto swallows and says, "Large, Doctor, but not so agreeable."

Asked about his diet, he tells about friends bringing big shrimp cocktails to his house. "So much, I ate and ate, and then I had to give the rest as a treat to my little dog," he says. "That spoiled thing. When I make myself a milkshake, she's always standing there watching me, so of course I have to give her her portion of it too."

"What's your dog's name?" I ask.

"Super."

Don Alberto is taking AZT and is getting interferon injections with it.

Russell asks him where he got his sun. "In my orchard. I was out there working. If I don't do anything, then my muscles ache, so I get up and work."

Russell goes out.

"What kinds of things do you have in your orchard?" I ask.

"It's really only about ten trees," Don Alberto says, "lemons and oranges, all kinds of things."

He is a widower. He contracted the virus and gave it to his wife. She became ill and died, but Don Alberto remains relatively healthy.

In the middle of the next client's time, Russell's nurse comes in, followed by a woman I have seen upstairs with the patient Juanito. Not his mother, though. There is a crisis, she says. This morning they brought Juanito down for X rays, and he's still in there, very sick.

"I'll come in a just a little bit, señora," Russell promises.

He finishes with the present client and then another, then gets up suddenly to go around and see what's happening in X Ray.

The corridor is deserted, dark. Nothing but the sound of the rain and the birds calling. Russell tries the first of two doors in a long wall of opaque glass, but it's locked. He is knocking on the second and calling to be let in when I notice Juanito's mother sitting in a wheelchair in the shadows across from the doors. She is bundled up in a bulky rain-soaked coat, her long thick gray hair wet and straggly down her back.

Inside, consternation. Technicians in their "whites," the big shiny gray X-ray machine. The air conditioning is blasting away and it is freezing in here. Juanito lies on his side on the metal table under the huge camera not talking, not moving, curled up like a great bird. There is pink stuff, the barium solution, all over his mouth and his thin gown. Russell speaks to him, but Juanito doesn't respond. Without turning, Russell asks no one in particular, "How long has this man been down here?" The staff doesn't know. An hour? More? They confer among themselves.

The third floor, 12:30 P.M. By the time Russell finishes his rounds, Juanito's x rays have come up. I hold them in place up against the staff room window for him while Russell solicits opinions from the other doctors. The pictures are good, they all agree. Upper and lower GI. "Here, at a half-hour, at two hours." What they show, though, seems to be no more than what Russell has already told me, that everything in Juanito's intestinal tract is blocked up. Russell admits to the others he doesn't know what to do. They nod, don't say anything, turn to other business. "Should I just send him home?" Russell says to no one in particular.

I think of Don Alberto, the handsome, jolly man with the little dog and the fruit trees, as an "older gentleman," though we are the same age, fifty. He was a salesman before he retired.

Not really expecting an answer, I wonder aloud how he must feel about having given the disease to his wife. Alejandro says that Don Alberto's grown daughters claim their father spent all his considerable fortune on boys. He would always bring them home. Their mother knew about it. She'd go away to visit her family and he'd fill the house with them. From the time they were little girls, the daughters claim, they saw their father having sex with boys.

In the afternoon after José Manuel has gone and Russell has also left for the day, Alejandro sits working at his desk, smoking as he writes.

A tentative knock at the door and a big-boned young man comes into the office. His name is Josué (Joshua in English), and he has a terrible headache. He is very apologetic to Alejandro about it, but it's just driving him nuts, he says. Josué is cross-eyed, which at the moment makes it look as though he's possessed, trying to focus in on this awful event going on upstairs in his head. He has a scraggly beard and a shock of hair he keeps raking through his fingers, as if the action might help him get control over whatever is wrong. He is very restless.

Alejandro asks Josué to answer some questions:

"How old are you?"

"I am thirty-two."

"What's *my* name?"

"You are Dr. Guerrero."

"Good. And where are we right now?"

"In the IMSS clinic."

"What day is it?"

"Wednesday."

Alejandro decides to admit him right away. He writes out the order and sends Josué off with it.

"Are these migraines or neurological symptoms of the disease itself?" I ask.

Alejandro surprises me. "Or is it neurosis? I don't know yet."

Thursday morning during Russell's rounds, I find Josué sitting up in a bed on the third floor wearing a gown. "How's your head feel today?" I ask.

"All right," he says. Then he admits, "Actually, not much better." He is very sweet. He looks frightened and breathes in a shallow, hungry way.

Josué has big, thick feet which are encrusted with something. I can't tell whether it is a fungus (out of control athlete's foot, for example) or the way he was born or the result of working barefoot all his life.

Thursday morning the office receives a visit from a diminutive doctor in white T-shirt and white pants. He is all bulked up, maybe a weight lifter, and comes from Hunucmá, a town on the road northwest toward the port of Sisal. He tells us he will be giving a safe-sex talk to nurses in the clinic where he works and needs what he keeps referring to as "the information." José Manuel prepares a packet of brochures, rolls up some posters and secures them with a rubber band, and gets out a big box of condoms.

The little doctor is also interested in getting "information" about the VIH testing done here, what the hours are, how soon you get your results back. All the while José Manuel is stressing the confidentiality of the process, the doctor from Hunucmá feels along under his chin and onto the back of his neck where there are lymph nodes.

Later, seven or eight well-dressed and well-mannered fourteen- or fifteen-year-old boys troop in. They seem to be on some sort of school assignment. Standing in a semicircle around José Manuel's desk with their hands in their pockets, they listen relatively solemnly while he tells them that SIDA is a serious business, a matter of life and death, and gives each of them a pamphlet. Then he gets out the box of condoms and allows them to choose some and stuff them into their pockets. Seeing the group to the door, José Manuel says, "And if there's anything more we can do for you boys—" in a voice so husky with innuendo the boys blush and laugh.

Then, at about ten o'clock, Aurelio, the waiter from across the street, comes in to collect the soda bottles that belong to his restaurant. A lean man in his forties, from Campeche I think, he sits and takes a rest, his wipe-up rag still draped over his shoulder.

"What's your *comida* over there today?" Alejandro and Russell ask.

"Chicken in *mole*."

"Which *mole*?"

"The dark. Tomorrow," Aurelio says, "it's stuffed fillet of shark. They've bought the fish already and it's going to be good."

Sex education seems to be on everybody's mind today. Aurelio tells how a doctor came to his fourteen-year-old daughter's school this week to give them a lecture about SIDA. He and his wife are glad the girl now has the facts. They've never hidden things about sex from their children, he says. When something comes up in a drama on television, they take the opportunity to tell the children about it. One time recently, in one of the television *novelas*, a doctor got stuck with a needle from a SIDA patient and she died, quickly.

"Well," I say, "that's television."

"I know," Aurelio says. "I used to mess around some, but with this thing I've stopped it completely."

"Have you?"

He seems to have more to say, but I appear to be the only one listening, so he sighs, braces himself with his hands on his knees, and gets up and begins collecting the bottles in his arms.

Eleven o'clock rolls around, time for Jenny's birthday celebration. She was in earlier and promised to be here, but she hasn't returned yet.

The young *promotor* Hugo Vargas has been sent off to get the cake, which turns out to be a yellow multilayered sponge spread with lots of white icing and topped with colored icing flowers. A large pot of water is put on to boil, and while we are waiting we drink coffee. "Where is she?" Russell asks, drumming his fingers on the table. Alejandro is in and out. José Manuel has to do an errand, but he returns.

Eventually Jenny comes in, does a laugh and big eyes at the sight of the cake. The gentlemen sing "Happy Birthday" in English. Russell even knows the beginning of the second verse "Stand up, stand up—" but he peters out. Jenny cuts, serves big slices. Fresh water is put on for more coffee.

Once we start eating, the conversation turns to the baby to come. Everything makes Jenny blush, even the question of whether she thinks it's going to be a girl or a boy. Alejandro goes back to his work, Russell remembers something he has to do, the party begins to break up. Jenny starts to get out her typing materials, but Alejandro tells her it's her birthday, she can do all that next week.

Later, I thought how pleasant the little period had been while all the men sat waiting for the guest of honor. A breather. The complacent expectation of boys when there is cake in the offing.

My thought about Hugo Vargas had been that if Alejandro could find the money to employ him, someone as gentle and low-key as Hugo would be an excellent safe-sex educator for schools and for drop-ins at the SIDA office at the T-1. But Alejandro seems worried by the mystery of Hugo's just showing up, hanging around.

"Maybe he's a spy from Pro Vida," I say.

"Possibly," says Alejandro.

Finally, this afternoon he calls Hugo over to his desk, tells him he doubts there will be any work for him here any time soon. Hugo accepts the news calmly, nodding, saying, "Well—"

Ni picha, ni cacha . . . , according to José Manuel. That may be. But today, before quitting time, Hugo asks permission and then goes to the filing cabinet and fills the pockets of his *guayabera* with a whole string of silver-foil condoms. When he shows them to us, grinning and blushing, José Manuel and I ask if he thinks that will be enough to get him through the weekend.

They came in Thursday, two very dolled up young ladies, to make an appointment for their VIH test Friday. They took chairs, talked extremely politely to Alejandro. When they left, José Manuel asked Hugo if he could tell they were men.

"I wasn't sure," Hugo said, "until I heard their voices."

In the morning they are nervous. One has on a soft pleated dress with a wide rhinestone-studded belt worn loosely, hanging down. Her complexion is soft, her manner soft also. She goes first, handing her small purse with the long strap to her friend, pushing her sleeve up above her elbow. The other one has on a miniskirt and a tight, frilly blouse, a mass of black hair, pomped curls in the front, then pulled back tight and let fall down the back. Bright red lipstick, eyeliner. More of a tough, Madonna look than her friend, smooth chest emphasized by the low blouse, although I don't remember breasts especially.

Laughing, they admit that neither one of them likes the idea of blood or being stuck with things. The first one turns her head away and looks down and to the side before José Manuel inserts the needle under the skin inside her elbow, while her friend watches. When José Manuel presses the cotton swab on the puncture and shows her how to hold it in place, she lets out a sigh of relief. The other girl then gives her purse to the softer one, and also looks away. But there is less drama this time.

It's over. José Manuel asks them how old they are. One is named Inés, I think, the other's name I don't recall. Nineteen and twenty. The softer one is going to school to become a chef. José Manuel explains that they can come in for their result Monday or any morning next week and that no one outside the clinic will know their real names. Then he compliments them on having taken the care to get the test.

Oh yes, well, they say, casting it off a little, shrugging (it is also an admission of their being sexual), pleased with the attention and the compliment from the official source. They thank everybody, José Manuel, Alejandro, me—perfect ladies—and take their leave.

Later, I ask José Manuel if the one who is going to cooking school could pass. "What do you mean?" he says. "They are both passing."

"At a job, I mean."

"Sure, why not?"

He begins to reminisce about other *travestis*. Poor Juanito upstairs. Then about another guy who had a white VW bus, a "*combi*," which he used to load up with beer and boys, and then he'd say, "See you, everyone! *We're* going out to the beach to fuck."

"Come in!" Russell calls.

An unscheduled intrusion in the middle of Russell's busy Friday morning clinic. The nurse Magdalena has the patient Josué's older sister, a big-faced, good-looking woman with lipstick on. She bustles right in, addresses Russell. It seems the pills that her brother was given finally began working for his headaches. But then last night someone told him they were going to draw spinal fluid on him today, and he got all upset and nervous about that. Russell assures her that no such order was given. He doesn't know where that one came from. She's sent back upstairs to tell her brother—and the nurses.

A man in his late fifties, early sixties, called Don Francisco. Clean, simple clothes, a worn white shirt, blue pants, *huaraches*. He works at a cement plant on the north edge of Mérida, and he has a slip of paper to hand over to Russell. Russell explains the report means there is no typhoid fever to worry about.

"What?" Don Francisco seems not to understand.

Russell raises his voice. "What's it all about? I'm happy to be the one to tell you it was all about *nothing*, Don Francisco. You can go back to work, everything is fine!"

After Don Francisco shuffles out, Russell explains to me that this is only a referral. Not SIDA-related at all. Something showed up on a test that made someone think the man had typhoid fever, but he didn't.

Next, a man about thirty, flushed red complexion. He is wearing white leather sandals. Bernardo. He has been having diarrhea for three days and feels weak. Russell has him weigh himself. Down two and a half kilos from less than a week ago. Russell asks him does he still have candidiasis. Yes. Bernardo shows his tongue, which is all pasty white. Russell fills out the forms to admit him to the hospital.

Josué's sister returns to report her brother is now more nervous than ever. They *told* him they were going to take this spinal fluid from him, they *told* him.

"Now señora, exactly *who* said that?"

"The neurologist, they say it's the neurologist who put in the order."

"Wait here for me a minute. I'll go talk to the neurologist myself." And Russell stalks out.

The sister and I are both standing. Things are really bad at home, she tells me. It's just her little brother and her mother, who is so old she really can't even take care of herself anymore, much less look after

Josué. "I come by whenever I can. Every day. In fact, I'm nearly back living there again myself now. But I've got my own family to tend to as well, my daughters, and my poor brother's just so nervous all the time he can't sleep, he paces around, sometimes I think he's just out of his mind, you know."

She speaks in torrents of words, not hysterical, but relentless, reasonable sounding. With Russell not present, she talks to me. When I look down and avoid her eyes, she addresses Magdalena the nurse.

Russell comes back, sits. Very low-key, a sigh. "I spoke with the neurologist, señora, and there's no order, nothing to worry about. Here, take this." He dashes off something on a piece of paper and hands it to her. "I'll come up to see your brother as soon as I can."

She is satisfied. "Thank you, Doctor." She turns and also thanks me before she goes out.

What can life be like at Josué's house? Do they all hector one another like this all the time?

Are the families made to understand the mental confusion that may come with the illness? Russell says toxoplasmosis is widespread in the Yucatán because of the way people let their cats shit in their gardens and because of bird shit in the thatch of houses, even close in to the city.

The next visitor is *very* nervous. He bustles right in, sits right down, his leather briefcase upright on his lap. Plenty of rings, necklaces. Thinned out. Suffering from weight loss, he tells me. But today the problem is his work excuse, his *incapacidad de trabajo*, which has been incorrectly written. Talking rapidly, he fishes the paper out, hands it over, then bends over to stare at it upside down as Russell reads it, agrees, writes out a new version.

Then a little man, precise, young, in a clean pressed white shirt. He perches on his chair, takes off his sunglasses and hooks them into the V of his collar. (He reminds me suddenly of my own more usual life as a patient, how you prepare for the big moment with the doctor. What will today's headline be? What *don't* I want the doctor to know about me this time? Or ever? How to alarm him or charm him into finally paying my health the attention it needs. What to wear? Clean underwear, the shirt Ray insisted on ironing, though to me it looked fine before.) The present client has just recently started using AZT. The first week he had "colic" with it, he says, but now nothing, no headaches or anything. He doesn't understand whether he's supposed to go to Dr. Guerrero, who saw him first, or to come now to Dr. Rodriguez.

"How long ago did you take the test?" Russell asks.

"Nineteen eighty-seven. I've known since 1987."

"So why are you only starting the drug now?"

The young man in the white shirt looks at me, a little smile. "I thought, 'If one is going to die, then one is going to die.' "

"Well," Russell says, "if you come with me, you're going to have to go on living for a while. All right?"

"Yes. Are you upset with me, Doctor?"

"For what? How could I be upset? I'm the sweetest man in the world—"

Magdalena comes in. The "engineer" who called has dropped by and is waiting to see Russell. "Ah," says Russell, glancing at his watch, looking down at his listing of appointments, "another one not on the program."

He turns back to the guy in the white shirt. "My little daughter's friends say, 'Oh, aren't you afraid your papa's going to scold you?' but my daughter laughs and says, 'How could that be? *My* papa's the sweetest man in the world.' "

The engineer proves to be a big man in his forties in a *guayabera*. He pulls papers from his briefcase and hands them over to Russell. Russell asks me to help translate. One of the forms they're interested in seems to be a standard blood panel that a VIH-positive person might take, leukocytes, p24 antigens, and so forth. At first I think the engineer may be a private client, then that he must work in the IMSS system in some capacity or another. Then he brings forth several small injection bottles, which Russell examines—clear liquid—then puts in his pocket. Finally, he gives Russell a letter in English, two pages long, on the stationery of a doctor in one of the northern states of the country. The second page has a place for a signature. The engineer goes out to get something from his car, and Russell explains to me that the doctor in the north has a medicine he claims will wipe out the SIDA virus. "For people for whom there's no other hope," Russell says, "why not try it?" They want to test it, start treatment, and they've determined Mérida is a good site. Not like the border towns, easily available from Miami or Houston by plane, pleasant. The cost will be great—$10,000 to $40,000 a year. In addition to the elixir, there appears to be treatment with an extraction of your own body fluids, which are then mixed up into a specific "antiviral" by the doctor in the north himself.

A client named Lorenzo Mena, a wizened, small, fast-moving person in his late fifties. He's come for a prescription, a check-in, and it goes quickly. All three of us stand throughout the visit. Russell says, "Our Lorenzo here is keeping himself alive through magic and black witchcraft," which sends the little man off into cackling laughter.

(Later, when I asked José Manuel what Russell meant, he said, "Exactly what he said. Lorenzo is a man who was somewhat crazy even before he became VIH.")

We take a break, go back to the clinic office. The young man in the white shirt who put off beginning AZT all those years has left boxes of ladyfingers, one for José Manuel and one for Alejandro. Alejandro says we can have them with our coffee. We're out of *instante*, however, so I go across the street to the grocery store to buy more. Just as I'm finishing at the checkout counter, all the lights go out. Everyone sighs. Back at the T-1, the water in José Manuel's electric pot is only lukewarm. We wait. The new air conditioning unit has shut down too, of course, so the office begins to warm up. If there isn't going to be coffee, someone decides, then at least we can have Cokes. Hugo Vargas returns to the grocery to get them.

Juanito's mother comes in looking for Dr. Russell, but Russell has gone off to deal with another patient. Juanito's mother doesn't know where Russell's office is, so I walk her over there. The other patient, a young man, is just leaving. Juanito's mother says her son now *only* wants to go home to his own house, that he refuses to stay in the hospital.

"Who can care for him there?" Russell asks.

"Well," the señora says, "I can go over there sometimes, and *maybe* some of his friends will come by, but basically there isn't anyone. But he still wants to go."

"Well, all right," Russell responds calmly. "I can't hold him you know, and maybe it's for the best. I'll be right up."

Five or seven minutes and two clients later, Russell is suddenly ready to go make his rounds. We take the elevator to the third floor, pace along the corridor, me hurrying in his wake. Russell charges right into the SIDA patients' room and right up to Juanito's bed.

"All right, Juanito, what is this?"

"Please, Doctor, I just want to go home. I beg you, I plead with you."

"Well, you are free to go. Take a taxi, whenever you want to. But let's get one thing straight, Juanito. *I* am not going to release you. Who's going to take care of you?"

"Lupita—"

"The nurse here?"

"Yes. She's my friend, she's promised she'll come."

"Once. One shift a day. But what about the other two?"

Juanito's mother is standing on the far side of the bed. She starts to speak, but Juanito overrides her. "I'll find someone. Please, Doctor, I'm begging you. I can't stay alive here."

"And as a physician in good conscience I can't let you go. Look here, the medications you're on are difficult to administer. They are marked 'For Use Only in IMSS Hospitals.' They can't be released to patients. Even if your family or friends didn't complain, somebody else might see them, and I have no right to give them to you. Why *can't* you stay with me a while, Juanito? At least give me the chance to complete this particular course of medicine with you and clear up what you have now. Otherwise *I* don't have a chance."

And with that Russell turns and stalks toward the door, past the other patients, the women feeding their boys lunch, the startled staff. Before he can get out, though, Miguel's mother stops him. Miguel looks awful at the moment. He is taking an antibiotic intravenously that is so strong it makes him sweat and tremble and sometimes moan out loud. Both arms are encased from elbow to wrist in aluminum foil to keep them from being exposed to light. Russell gives a brief answer to Miguel's mother's question, then leaves.

I follow him out. He is standing in the center of the hall calling for nurses. When they don't appear immediately, he changes his tune. "Where are all the residents then? I need to talk with them." One comes scurrying along and Russell undertakes a reasonable discussion with him about what to do about Bernardo, the man with diarrhea he admitted earlier this morning.

Then he goes back into the room. Juanito is arguing quietly with his mother while she spoon-feeds him Jello. When he sees the doctor, he stops.

"Well, Juanito? What have you decided?"

Juanito says he will stay for a while. Clearly he is afraid to lose access to the medications he's taking. Likely also he doesn't want to lose Russell. Juanito speaks calmly, still very much in charge of himself. His agreement to endure another ten days in this place has the nature of a deal.

At three, as Alejandro, José Manuel, and I are getting ready to leave for the day, the patient Jorge Dario Valle's mother comes in to have a talk with José Manuel. With her is her daughter, also a nurse, who is wearing a tight IMSS-green skirt and a high-shouldered white blouse. I can see the resemblance between Jorge and his sister but not, in this case, between mother and daughter. I ask if I can sit with them, and draw up a chair. José Manuel introduces me. The mother nods, says she knows me from upstairs. She is wearing a *huipil* as usual, and small earrings. She is not much older than I, though freckled skin hangs loose under her arms and at her neck.

"Well, then," José Manuel says, his eye on the mother, "let's begin. Look, *mi reina*, we are at the point where I'm going to have to tell you a few things. And whenever I have to do this, I always wish that I didn't. But in the case of your son, we are all aware of what a great fight he has put up, and of how different he is now from the man he was a month ago when we first got the opportunity to come to know him. And I can tell you we all know that God is great, and it may be that our Jorge will still rise up again and we will see him returned to being the way we knew him. With God, as they say, everything is possible. But we also have to prepare ourselves for other possibilities. He doesn't have a lot of strength left in him, and he isn't getting any better. This thing has exhausted him."

Jorge Dario's mother's small bright eyes have clouded up and she has begun to weep silently.

José Manuel says, "Now don't cry, señora, because I can assure you—and you know this is true—that those of us here have done and are going to continue to do precisely nothing less than the most we possibly can do for your son. And if God takes him, then we have to have faith that God wants our Jorge for *His* purposes. But you know, he may just come back to us and rise up again tomorrow."

Now the sister is crying also. José Manuel puts his hand over the mother's hand and pats it. I think *I* may start crying, too, but I look

José Manuel right in the face and see he's going to remain dry-eyed, so with some effort I am able to follow his example.

Jorge Dario's mother stands up, the tears running down her cheeks, and she and her daughter embrace.

In José Manuel's rattletrap old car a few minutes later he tells me that, being a nurse, Jorge Dario's sister understands everything about her brother's situation, but she hasn't been able to bring herself to tell any of it to her mother.

José Manuel has gotten me invited to the Friday night meeting of a new VIH support group he has helped organize. The six men who could come tonight are all in their thirties. We sit on couches and uncomfortable straight-back dining room chairs around a cheap laminated coffee table in the ground-level condo a man named Horacio shares with his lover. The lover, in cutoffs and T-shirt, is in and out, sometimes perched listening on a stool at the eating bar, sometimes in the back of the house.

They begin by introducing themselves to me: Horacio, who has a military sort of bearing (he works in security), says that he and his lover are "working things out"—the questions that come from him being positive and his lover negative. Still completely asymptomatic, he says. He points out that the group is largely homosexual, but not necessarily gay pride. José Manuel is brief. "Everyone knows me," he says. "Nineteen years old, of course," for which he gets a laugh. "VIH." Then soft-spoken, sweet Rubén, whom I already know, and Fernando, a thinned-out, quiet blond man with blue eyes, wearing a red and white striped polo shirt, who mentions he's already had "both social problems and medical problems." Then Pedro, who says he's experienced some weight loss, that's all. He had a big career in politics, economics, managed large government factories in the north—the last one had sixteen thousand workers. When he found out he was VIH-positive, he figured he needed to simplify his life and calm down, so he moved to Mérida, where he does a less stressful version of the work he used to do.

The member of the group newest to the single great knowledge they all share is Adalberto, "Beto" for short. A thickset man with receding hair, rimless glasses, jeans, a plain short-sleeve white shirt, he is still healthy, he says. Beto only learned about what he calls his "status" three months ago. It came as a big surprise to him, since he and his lover very seldom did anything outside their relationship. He is from an oil-boom town in the state of Tabasco. There was hepatitis in his family, so he went to take a blood test. "I was crushed when I found out," he tells the others. "In the beginning I didn't know whether I was going to make it to Christmas Eve." Now there's trouble between him and his partner, and he doesn't know what will come of it. He has high expectations of this group, Beto says.

Almost all the others present belonged to an earlier support group that fell apart. They nod when José Manuel mentions that "unfortunately" someone made off with the old group's treasury and decide this time to take up a collection and to give one another chits until they have more or less equaled out the expenditures. On the question of what to name themselves ("War and Peace" and "Positive Life" are suggestions) they cannot get a consensus, so they put off the question for the next week.

By now it is eleven o'clock, and I am not the only one with a big case of the yawns. In conclusion, they ask if I have any advice for them. What to say? They seem fully efficient and mobilized on the organizational front, but except for Beto in one brief flash, all evening they've been stepping quite carefully to avoid getting into anything where their own emotions are involved. So I recall Rubén, who talked earlier about there not being psychologists in Mérida willing to help people like them. Maybe having just themselves will turn out to be an advantage, I say, give them the possibility of doing something entirely new, of confronting problems together. "Don't forget what a resource you can be to one another. If the world doesn't approve of us, then we will approve of ourselves."

They thank me profusely and tell me I'll be their mascot and that I am welcome to come visit them whenever I'm around.

After the meeting four of us go back into the center of town to a new gay nightclub called "Papaya." Pedro hesitates about going in. Any chance of the police, a *redada*? No, no, José Manuel assures him, everything's paid off. To get in costs 20,000 pesos (almost U.S. $7.00) and includes a couple of very weak drinks and eventually a "show" staged on a large platform in the middle of a columned courtyard open to the night sky. A singer adds his own pleasant-enough voice to a prerecorded orchestra mix of "Cuatro Caminos," and then two boy go-

go dancers strip to disco songs, gyrating into standard muscle poses. They never get further down than their posing straps, and the applause for them is half-hearted.

Well after midnight, music for dancing begins. For a while no one gets up. Then a pair of older men venture onto the platform. Pedro and Beto dance. Rubén and I. José Manuel comes up a couple of times, but only when asked. I sit with him and we hold hands and kiss some. Up on the stage Beto, who seemed so depressed earlier in the evening, is getting into it. He comes down for a gulp of his drink, wipes his forehead with his pocket handkerchief. I ask if he is ready to go again. He is. We dance to a long sequence of Madonna songs, followed by fifties and sixties rock 'n' roll. Beto shakes his butt earnestly, a kind of rolling, latinized twist step.

Though the night air is cool, I am sweating. I am also pleasantly drunk. I sit next to José Manuel again, hand on his neck in the back of his green jersey, and tell him what a wonderful job I thought he did this afternoon informing Jorge Valle's mother about her boy's condition. "I thought I was going to cry," I say, "but then I thought, 'What is there for *you* to cry about right now? This isn't your thing. Don't intrude on it.' "

"I was going to cry too," José Manuel admits. Then he does, weeping and weeping, and I put my arm around him and he goes on, muffled, against my chest. Coming up for air, he says, "It's the kind of thing neither Russell or Alejandro can do. Or at least they won't. So I always have to do it."

It's 3:00 A.M. when we finally leave the Papaya. In the dead, silent street we exchange big *abrazos* all around.

"It was good to see you dance," I tell Beto.

"Oh, I love dancing," he says. "But this is the first time I've done it since I found out about my status."

Alejandro has been sent a copy of a letter written by the sister of a man who was a school teacher on the island of Cozumel. The man and his wife, also a school teacher, are both VIH-positive. In translating the letter, I have left the sentences as they are, ending mostly with commas, and have tried also to maintain the sister's formal, bleak style:

Cozumel Quintana Roo, 19 February 1992
C. Dr. Javier Ramírez Nava
Director of the ISSSTE Clinic in Cozumel
Quintana Roo

Señor director, by means of the present I want to register my complaint against Dr. —, a doctor in your clinic, since he has consistently dealt badly with my brother, Professor —, who it seems now carries the illness known as SIDA, according to the doctor my brother can no longer travel by bus or airplane to the city of Chetumal, because he would infect the passengers, the doctor even told me my brother ought not be admitted to the ISSSTE [clinic] because of the possibility that *he* or the nurses or the other patients hospitalized there could become infected by being in contact with my brother, he also told me that my brother *and my sister-in-law* would be confined in Mérida and not allowed to leave, he also told me that even my mother and I would have to take an examination since surely we are also infected, and even if we ran off to Chetumal they would track us down there in order to make us take this examination, moreover he stated that my brother had had sex with a homosexual and that *he* was the chief source of the infection. Dr. Ramirez, I beg your consideration because my family does not know what to do, and even if what Dr. —(if he *is* any sort of a doctor) says is true I believe there exist more professional and educational means for conveying these things. I send you this letter knowing you to be a person of good judgment. Please, Doctor, help us as much as possible in the cause of my brother's illness. Attentively, —

Alejandro says the poor school teachers were in a restaurant talking, and the woman who is head of the Cozumel chapter of the conservative national organization called Padres de Familia was sitting behind them and overheard their conversation. She got them thrown out of their jobs, and they fled down the coast to Chetumal. The wife is now sick enough so that she wouldn't be able to return to work, but the man would be perfectly capable of continuing at his job if they would let him.

José Manuel's car stalls out and dies in traffic. Luckily, the car is light enough and turns over easily enough so that he can often get it started again by pushing it himself. Alejandro's current vehicle is also a wreck. The window on the passenger side won't roll up and the door can only be opened from inside. Tonight I notice that a stack of SIDA information on the floor by my feet has been turned into a soggy mass by Wednesday's showers.

Alejandro starts telling me about another client. I met her the other day when she came by to visit, a tall, blond woman in her late twenties from one of the states in the north. In 1985 or 1986 she had plastic surgery to reform her nose and became VIH-infected from a blood transfusion. Now she has a three-year-old son who is not positive, and her husband, a Yucatec, rejects her completely. She lives for her child, Alejandro says.

It makes her nervous to be seen at the clinic, so Alejandro goes out with her to talk, have a cup of coffee. "Really all I can do is listen to her," he says. "She is one of those people with a lot of problems and no one to tell them to. We've become as close as it's possible to be without breaking the doctor-patient relation."

"Have you talked with the husband?"

"He doesn't want to deal with it."

"Have you tried talking to them together?"

"One time. But the husband has never come back."

One possibility, I say, is that the man still loves his wife and can't stand to think about what is going to happen to both of them. If this is the case, there are *two* tragedies in operation at the same time, hers facing death and his facing the "possibility" (the certainty) that she is going to leave him. That he hasn't left her yet may well mean that he does still love her and is suffering the loss to come in silence.

"With a succession of other women, actually," Alejandro says.

Then, as though the thought is connected, Alejandro tells me his own father, in his eighties now and long retired from the Air Force, has been having heart attacks and won't survive long. He and Alejandro's mother live in their retirement in Michoacán.

It is also the evening Alejandro tells me, "I don't really know what led me to this practice, but it has made my life for me."

Sunday morning I go to the T-1 about ten to meet Alejandro on the third floor, but he is late. Bernardo, the young man admitted Friday for diarrhea, is hanging out in the hall in his blue gown and white sandals.

We shake hands and I follow Bernardo back into the SIDA patients' room.

The medication has caused a drastic improvement in Miguel's condition. The IV and the oxygen have disappeared from the head of his bed, the spooky coverings of aluminum foil are gone from his arms, and his father, sporting a cap with "Captain" on the brim, has brought a wheelchair to take his son for a ride down the corridor and downstairs to get some fresh air. His mother stays to tidy up.

Jorge Dario Valle is fully awake, lying nearly nude in his bed. Yesterday he was wetting himself and they kept changing his sheets, but now they've put a catheter in. There is talcum powder on his thin white chest. His wrists are tied to the bed frame with gauze, but his good leg keeps straining up, lifting and waving, and I wonder if he's going to pull his tube out. No nurses are around. When I take Jorge's right hand, which is the side that's not paralyzed, he holds mine strong.

Josué, the man with the headaches, has gone home, and Juanito has been moved in one bed from the window. He is sleeping, hooked up to an IV. Very thin, his long hands folded over his chest. I talk some with Bernardo, touch his warm back where his gown opens. He is wearing a black digital wristwatch. The vomiting has stopped, he says, and the diarrhea is down to a couple or three times a *torno* (shift).

Jorge Dario slowly reaches his stockinged foot up to the table across the bottom of his bed and touches an apple.

"What's he trying to do?"

"He wants his apple," Bernardo says. "But he'd have to eat it in pieces and there aren't any knives around."

On his table there's a tangerine. "Do you think he'd like this?"

No one seems to know.

I peel the tangerine and remove some sections, taking out the seeds and as much of the stringy pulp as I can. Jorge Dario opens his mouth and takes the sections off my fingers, one by one. He chews mildly, opens his lips for more. When he's done he sighs and says in English, "*Tank yoo very much.*"

After the meeting with Alejandro, I come back in to say my goodbyes. Juanito is awake. A new tube protrudes from his abdomen. He has already filled half a bottle with the brown liquid from his intestines.

"How are you, Juanito?"

"Not good," he says. "I feel awful." He takes my hand. "What am I going to do?"

"What do you mean?"

"I want so much to be out of this place and in my own house. I really don't want to live any more, you know."

I stroke his long beautiful hand. There is clear polish on his nails. Finally I say, "How old are you?"

"Thirty-one."

"And you've accomplished a lot—"

"Yes, I have." He looks toward the window. "The man I loved—" He pauses, then says, "I don't know how to get in touch with him, and I only pray to God that he doesn't have this same thing and doesn't have to suffer the way I have."

"How long have you had it?"

He doesn't answer. So I say, "José Manuel told me all about your singing, your performances."

"Oh yes—"

"I wish I could have heard you."

"I wish you could have too. Do you believe in Heaven?"

"Well—in a way."

He says, "I do. In Heaven, but not in another life. I don't want one."

I have my hand laid on his bony forehead when he says something and my Spanish fails me. I think maybe he wants me to kiss him. I lean close in and Juanito says, "I would like your blessing."

It seems too complicated at the moment to tell him I'm not sure I have a blessing to give. So I say, "You can have that."

A nurse appears with a big syringe. She is about to inject it into Juanito's arm but he says something and she goes away without doing anything to him.

"You know I'm going tomorrow, Juanito."

"I heard that."

"But I'll look for you, whether it's here or over there."

"All right," he says. "Good."

THE CAPTAIN'S TOUCH

Chamula, the Chiapas *municipio* where I was first sent in 1963, had a reputation for being inhospitable to outsiders. As far as I could tell, other than the ladino secretary and the government employees who slept in dormitories in the town center, in the previous twenty-five years only three other non-Indian people had been allowed to move about the community with relative freedom. One was the Mexican anthropologist Ricardo Pozas, another Eric Prokosh, a fellow Harvard Chiapas Project student. The third had been Ruth Bunzel, best known for her ethnography of Chichicastenango in Guatemala. Trained at Columbia University by Franz Boas, Bunzel was, with Margaret Mead and Ruth Benedict, a member of a famous anthropological triumverate known as "the Boaz girls."

But Bunzel had spent only three months in Chamula in 1940, and published only one article from her fieldwork there. When I asked why she had stayed so short a time, my professors said the *story* was that she had been run out for going around at night with a flashlight trying to find out about the Indians' sex lives.

I have no idea whether the flashlight tale is true. I tend to think it is mostly gossip, but whether gossip perpetrated by her colleagues in anthropology or by tongue-waggers among the Maya I cannot tell. (A man in Zinacantán, the town next to Chamula, has the nickname "The Flashlight," because he is said to use one to watch himself and his wife have intercourse.) What I *do* know is the puzzlement the story caused me and some of the other students in my cohort. I remember discussing the matter with Shelly Zimbalist, who ended up going on to become an anthropologist just about the time I decided not to. To us the obvious implication of the flashlight story was that there was something déclassé about sex research itself. Not a subject for the career-mindful.

Yet we were confused. Anthropology then still had its popular reputation for being highly concerned, if not obsessed, with sex. Mead, Benedict, Malinowski, the best-known people in the field, all had achieved fame writing about sexuality in other cultures. But the generation that included our teachers, while not particularly prudish personally, studied subjects like the intricacies of kinship and numeral classifiers, models of acculturation and the names for different kinds of firewood. The second summer we were in Chiapas together, Shelly interviewed Zinacantec men and women on their concepts of the human body, a subject she then used to cross over into discussing beliefs about sex and sexuality. No one prohibited her work; in fact she was encouraged to do it. But as far as I can tell, she never wrote up any of it for publication.

Today, every graduate student knows that fashions and cultural imperatives of the anthropologists' own society strongly influence what they will write about others. In those days we were not so sophisticated and did not link the renewed repression in the United States following World War II with the apparent disdain for the subject of sex in American anthropology of the 1950s and 1960s. The Malinowski-Mead-Benedict generation had been self-conscious about being moderns. They thought a clear-headed recital of the facts about sex in other societies would cause their own to shrug off the remaining elements of Victorian prudery. (Alfred Kinsey had the same impulse, I think.) In the McCarthy period, when homosexuality was freely equated with traitorous disloyalty to the nation, the program of the "moderns" was put on hold and the discipline closed ranks over its own more various, more deviant past. The bisexuality of some of the leading figures and the homosexuality of others, once open secrets, were hushed up. And though social anthropology continued to attract and promote women as few other academic disciplines did, a version of cold war macho became the dominant style in the field. (In some ways, I think the story of Ruth Bunzel's flashlight may really be an allegory about why certain talented people from the 1920s and 1930s—women—never achieved the prominence or the positions they should have.)

The thaw did not come until the 1970s, when the new feminism and the gay/lesbian movements contributed to making sex and sexuality legitimate subjects to study again. The appearance of AIDS a few years later almost immediately made it obvious that, far from being obsessed with sex and sexuality, the anthropologists had been so negligent of the subjects that their accounts contained almost no data that could be useful in slowing the spread of the disease.

I thought of calling this chapter "Ruth Bunzel's Flashlight" to invoke this probably mythical object and let it serve as the sign under which the following three inquiries were conducted.

Eddie's Nail Scissors

DECEMBER 1988–MARCH 1990

I landed back in Mérida for the first time in twelve years knowing only one person I could still get in touch with. Bill Ballantyne had been a graduate anthropology student at Stanford in the sixties, then had married a Mayan woman and settled here, establishing an orchard and wholesale nursery on a piece of land outside the city limits. Bill was leaving the next day for Canada, so we only had one evening together. I told him my new plan—to try to learn what I could about AIDS and homosexuality in the Yucatán. There *was* AIDS here, he said, he had seen articles in the *Diario*. He also remembered that in Yucatec Maya one term for a homosexual was the word for a crab. Why, though, he could not figure, unless the reference was to the skittering, sideways movement of both. Otherwise, he said he didn't know anything much. When I asked whom I might talk with, the only person he could come up with was a businessman everyone calls *Don* Eddie.

About 9:00 P.M., shop closing time, we went around to "Eddie's Curios" and asked to speak with the gentleman himself. I recognized Eddie as soon as he came bustling out from his office in the back, a wiry little man in polo shirt and shorts, fifty-six, hair still black, hairy arms and legs as well, body holding together. He had begun his gift shop in this huge old downtown house on Calle 56, using first the downstairs and then expanding into the rooms off the courtyard balcony as he could afford to renovate them. Eddie's Curios had already been well established the first time I came to Mérida in the summer of 1963. Later, through contacts he made with gringo patrons, helping them find rental housing, Eddie had become heavily involved in real estate and, everyone says, very rich. Now, over the brandies with ice he brought out to us on the patio, his talk was about his place in the country, his orchards, the nightmare of having condos as well as the new shop to manage in Cancún at the same time he felt it necessary to be here at every moment because, except for his sister, there was no one he could trust to manage the Mérida operations in his absence. In recent years Eddie has set up a catering business with his brother-in-law. It also is run largely out of the old house. They do work for the country clubs, weddings, and the elaborate presentation parties for teenage girls called *quinceneras*, as well as most of the events at the Club Libanese.

Over time, Eddie has made an international set of friends, whom he gets to visit on sumptuous vacations. He mentioned Key West, Maui, Lake Tahoe, and then told about being given a private tour of the Las Vegas mansion of the famous lion tamers Siegfried and Roy. Eddie seemed to assume Bill and I would both already be well aware that the two performers were no longer an "item," and went about explaining how their vast place was now meticulously split into two completely separate camps, with only the mammoth swimming pool standing between them as a kind of indivisible "no man's land."

After about an hour we thanked Eddie, shook hands all around, and took our leave. Outside on the street, Bill was surprised at how reticent I had been. "Did you get what you wanted?" he asked.

"It was fine," I told him.

A couple of days later, around noon, I went by the shop again. A widow from San Diego was there to get Eddie's advice about beach houses to rent out in Progreso. The problem was that most of the usually available places had been destroyed in Gilbert, the great hurricane that had raked the peninsula in October. After a while, a couple of other older gringos, residents, started paying some attention to the San

Diego lady, and I asked Eddie if I could take up ten or fifteen minutes of his time. Of course, he said, as though he had been expecting it. He brought coffee from the back of the house and ushered me into a room full of shelves of pottery, much of it in need of dusting. I sat at a counter and Eddie stood behind it, stirring a sugar cube into his coffee. I started a half-prepared speech, but as soon as I got to the part concerning what *might* be done about SIDA in a place like Mérida, Eddie stopped me.

There *wasn't* anything to be done, he said. He himself had gotten the word a long time ago and had just stopped having sex. SIDA was just too much. These days, just the thought of sex would keep it limp. "Oh," he said then, reconsidering, "a year ago there was a guy, an Italian. We went upstairs and jacked off because *he* seemed to want it so much. But otherwise, no, not me."

Would he tell me more or less how sex between men was accomplished here?

He was ironic with me: "You don't know?"

"No, I'm completely ignorant."

"Oh, the gay men drive by in their cars and they say 'Want to go for a ride?' And the boy says no, he doesn't want to, so the man says, 'Oh come on, I'll just buy you a drink or a meal.' And the boy goes, and after the third drink the man says, 'Just let me see it,' or 'Just let me touch it,' and the boy takes it out and after the fourth drink he lets the man suck it and then maybe he fucks the man, or gets fucked himself even, and there's no rubber or anything and the boy swears to himself he'll never do *that* again, but three or four days later of course he's back out on that same street corner."

"Is that because the news isn't getting out?"

"Oh no, the news is all over the place, on posters, on walls, in the newspapers, on television. The mothers got all upset about that one, for them showing a condom on television. Or maybe it was for talking about sex, I don't remember."

"Are there condoms available?" I asked.

"In every drug store," Eddie nodded. "But no one uses them."

"And the Catholic Church? What does the Church here say?"

Eddie exploded. "No sex before marriage and that's it!" He looked at me, then in English said, "What do you care what they do, how many of them get AIDS? Me, I watch out for myself."

I tried to defend myself. Maybe as *older* people, we could be of help in some way.

"They'll never listen," Eddie said. "I was in Key West. There they see people your age and my age coming and all they can think anymore is 'AIDS, AIDS.' They cross the street to avoid us. And you know, I don't blame them one bit."

He wasn't finished. "And don't try to come on like you're down here to educate either. They don't need that, they don't even want to hear it. And don't preach those things to the gays. You were doing them yourself at that age, weren't you? So how can you tell *them* not to?"

"What about you, Eddie? Were you active as a kid?"

He laughed. "From the time I was twelve years old. Doing everything I could think of. Sitting waiting in the back of movie theaters to see who'd come along and suck my cock."

"Is there anything like a gay community in Mérida?"

"There used to be," Eddie said. "Just a bitchy bunch, but they had their parties and everything. I used to go, but I've stopped. Who needs people like that?"

"And is there anybody who is public and 'out' about it?"

"Are you kidding? Nobody would be such a fool. Even if they were all alone in the world, still they'd have mothers and sisters or nephews and they could never ever be open about it. Not in this town."

Eddie's estimate was that there had been about eight or ten AIDS deaths already in Mérida. People who thought they had it found themselves private doctors, and then when they died they got false death certificates listing the cause of death as heart attack or whatever.

Two gringos had had a guest house in town, he told me. Both of them died of SIDA, and then the people from Public Health came in and shut the place down. But now it was open again, he thought.

"Who's running it?"

"Oh, the houseboy they were fucking or whoever."

Then Eddie began to calm down. "What is it you still *could* do?" he wondered. "With your fingers maybe? But when I go out to my ranch and work with my hands, I get cuts all over them. What am I going to do?" He laughed. "Wear gloves?"

I told him I thought it unlikely you could get it from cuts on your hands.

Eddie had said that to learn about SIDA I needed to get in touch with Dr. Góngora at the Noguchi Center out by the University of Yucatán Medical School. Renán A. Góngora-Biachi turned out to be a small, round, friendly hematologist in his mid- to late thirties who worked mornings on research at the Center for Regional Investigations "Dr. Hideyo Noguchi" on Avenida Itzáes next to the O'Horán, which is Mérida's charity hospital. In the afternoons he had a practice across town at the fashionable Centro Médico Las Americas. The building that housed the department of hematology was run down, nineteenth- or very early twentieth-century, painted bright yellow outside. Inside, the hallways were dusty, the ceilings high above lost in cool gloom. A line of plastic-back chairs were set up for patients in the passage before you got to Góngora's own tight windowless office. The doctor's eyeglass case bore the name Gucchi, and there was a bottle of J&B scotch on top of the filing cabinet, together with cassettes of Disney cartoons. The cups and pens and desk calendars were the ones the drug companies give away.

Dr. Góngora did not discover the first cases of SIDA in the Yucatán, but he seems to have been the first to report on them in journal articles. The first two patients, who were diagnosed in 1983, were both homosexuals who had spent considerable time in the United States, he told me. The disease was thus an "import" to Yucatán. All the early cases were in men with means, but since then, as Dr. Góngora put it, SIDA has spread "downward" to other sorts of people. By the end of 1988, when I first talked with him, out of a population of about 800,000, 54 men and 2 women in Mérida had gotten SIDA. Two cases had been children, who were exposed through blood transfusions. The infection of the women Góngora thought had come from bisexual men, the women's husbands or lovers. The southeast of Mexico might well follow what he called "the African model," in which prostitutes would infect heterosexual men. His estimate was that ten thousand of the forty thousand homosexual men in Mérida might be seropositive. (The forty thousand figure he took from the census, using the assumption that all unmarried male heads of household over thirty must be homosexual.)

Góngora's general model for homosexual transmission was a story of wealthy gays becoming infected abroad, and then when they came home passing the virus to the young working-class men and boys they preyed on. An alternative route would be through the international gay tourists coming to Cancún and infecting local boys there. He mentioned a study (I think from Brazil) in which twenty-six hundred working-class men were surveyed and only four were found to be seropositive—all of them *albañiles* (masons, plasterers). Why that profession? I asked. Unskilled men from the country, the doctor said, working long hours on the outskirts of a city, themselves unsophisticated, uneducated, paid off every week at the job site—an easy place to be picked up by homosexuals.

Dr. Góngora and his research group had administered a questionnaire to a group of sixty-one homosexuals (three of these were referred medically, the others had answered an advertisement in the newspaper) and to male students in high schools. The adult homosexuals estimated that 85 percent of school-age boys in Mérida had had some kind of homosexual relations. The adolescents guessed that 35 percent of other boys had, but only 5 percent said that they themselves had had such relations.[1]

"Among themselves or with adults?"

"Both," Dr. Góngora said.

The group he was involved with (two of the doctors were homosexual, he said) concentrated on educating students and prostitutes about SIDA. They gave talks in schools, followed by frank question-and-answer sessions. The prostitutes were contacted through the Centro de Salud office in Mérida which tests and treats them for venereal disease. I asked whether his group was training college students to give the talks about SIDA, and Góngora said no, in fact they were increasing the number of doctors making the presentations. They found that people responded better to the authority of a medical person. He thought public meetings a better way than giving out pamphlets. Even the factories in the city were now beginning to invite speakers from his group.

I told the doctor I was interested in whether Mayan people were finding out about the disease, and asked did he think there was SIDA infection in the Mayan towns.

"Minimal," said Góngora.

The articles he gave me, both the scientific ones and those from the *Diario de Yucatán*, the state's most prominent and conservative newspaper, indicated that Dr. Góngora would prefer abstinence as a main educational message concerning SIDA. His understanding of homosexuality seemed to me quaint, and his models of transmission to require a class of careless gay villains blithely spreading SIDA among the innocent. But still, I appreciated the time he had given me and his politeness. When I got back to California, I wrote to thank him, let him know I was homosexual, and, since he had said he was coming to San Francisco, invited him to give a talk at my university. I didn't hear back from Dr. Góngora, but then I hadn't expected to.

After midnight there were boys on every corner around the Zócalo. There were also some along Calle 60 and up toward the park in Santa Lucia, but more in the main square, waiting around in T-shirts and jerseys, prefaded jeans, moving half a block up, returning. Not saying anything to each other if they passed. Downtown was quiet at last, the thundering rushes of the cars and trucks along the narrow streets at a cease. The last buses for the outlying colonias had left, and an acrid, dirty haze hung over everything.

One night around midnight I tried "Los Charros" at 60th and 53rd. A close and loud little place, it cost about U.S. $7.00 to get in. Kids, boys sixteen or seventeen, were hanging around the side street entrance, probably waiting for someone they knew to show up and pay their admission. It was very dark inside and there wasn't much of an audience for the little drag show they put on, half a dozen men in their fifties or sixties at tables with boys in their teens. The other *travestis* were not very good at their lip-syncing, but the M.C.. was a guy with a funny, fat little body—the shape of a juicy roasting chicken. He came out all bundled up in a beret and raincoat and sang an "intro" ("I'm sad as I walk along the boulevard of life," etc.) and then suddenly off came the raincoat and the beret, revealing him in a sequined singlet and ratty mesh stockings, and he was strutting up and down and singing away about the joys of being the "queen of the show." His patter had funny stuff about his mother helping him with his costumes and about what a bore it was being picked up all the time by the police. "I say, 'What's the problem, señores?' and they say, 'You're a transvestite!' And I say, 'That's right. What's the problem, señores?' "

Though I was pleased with what I had learned from Don Eddie and from Dr. Góngora, I also felt deflated. At times it seemed everything relevant was already known—both about AIDS/SIDA and about male homosexuality—and that nothing remained for me to learn about these hardly salient topics. Then, unexpectedly, some move, a gesture or a joke, would make me feel again that my "subject" was around me all the time, demanding attention.

One example: Because I had booked my ticket late, I was going back to the States by way of Cancún. To get across the peninsula, I rented a VW. Coming into Cancún, traffic was held up by construction and I had to sit and wait. By the side of the road were three young workmen with no shirts on, joking about something. One of them came up behind the other, grabbed him at the elbows, and began humping on his ass. The second man bent over a little and wiggled, as though he was enjoying being fucked. All three were laughing, apparently unconcerned about me and the other stalled drivers watching them.

David Muna was another man I had met in 1988 who I thought might be gay. When I came back to Mérida in the spring of 1990, I went to see him.

David sits most of the day on a stool, with his telephone on the counter beside him, polishing things and making little "fixes" in earrings and necklaces with needle-nose pliers. His reading glasses sit low on his nose. Glancing up, he can see whoever is going by or stopping to look at the jewelry display trays in his window. On shelves behind him are some brass dishes and Mayan figurines in reconstituted turquoise. Although he speaks English very well, David seems to sell mainly to local people, not tourists.

He was born in Mérida, is about fifty now, big, shoulders a little hunched, balding, deep-voiced. When I first met him, he was living with his mother at her house in the center of town. Now, fifteen months later, he announced that he had finally taken an apartment of his own and was cooking for himself, although usually he still went over to eat the main meal with his mother in the afternoons. On her back patio David's mother had *chinas* (eating oranges), which he sold for her in the park at Santa Lucia on Sundays. He was a writer of stories and songs, he told me, and had lived in Mexico City for various periods of time, mostly in pursuit of someone to publish his music. He had been to New York and had visited Guatemala. We talked once about how pretty Panajachel and Lake Atitlán were.

Alone with him in his shop, I mentioned having interviewed Renán Góngora-Biachi when I was in Mérida over a year ago. "Oh he's the worst," David said, "anti-gay, like a—," he had to shift into English to express it, "—a redneck."

Like Don Eddie, he dwelled on the story of the two gay men with the guest house over in the part of town sometimes called Gringo Gulch. David didn't know whether they were a couple, maybe just business partners. But anyway, it was parties every night—alcohol, drugs, pornographic movies—and "all the little Mayas from the plaza" would attend. In David's version, only one of the men got SIDA and died. The other? David didn't know what happened to him. Either he died or he went away—he must have been infected too. "The point is," he said, "who knows how many other people were infected through this one couple?"

I asked about boys coming out of the villages. "Oh yes," David said, "the carpenters and *albañiles* who work in Cancún, they get high wages, and *they* all come from other places. But when they get drunk they lose their money or they're robbed—do you know that everyone who lives in Cancún carries a gun at night? you have to—well, then some of them are bound to let their pants down (*bajar los pantalones*) in exchange for some cash or the price of a couple of beers."

Valladolid, halfway across the peninsula, is the second city in the state. David sniffed at the people there. "They're all so proud because there aren't any cases of SIDA reported yet in Valladolid. But I say, 'Where do the carpenters and the *albañiles* who are building Cancún come from? From towns like Valladolid, for sure.' "

In David's opinion what Mexico should have done from the beginning was give incoming tourists a blood test—and if the result came back positive, they shouldn't have been admitted. He also thought underreporting of cases was widespread in Mexico because doctors didn't always have the knowledge needed to recognize SIDA when it appeared. And he was aware that condoms are not 100 percent effective.

"Are they available here?"

"In any pharmacy." David looked up at me over his glasses. "But, of course, the ones here might be small for a man as big as you," he said, grinning.

A friend stopped in, a man in his fifties named Reinaldo Burgos, thin, good-looking, wearing a gold wedding ring. David told me

Reinaldo worked at a bank in town, and Reinaldo said, in English, "But not for much longer. In two years I get to retire." Next month Reinaldo was going to France to visit an Algerian-Spanish friend of his. I asked what the friend in France did, and Reinaldo said something about *tratante de blancas*.

After he left, I admitted to David that I had no idea what *tratante de blancas* means. "Whores," David said in English, "the guy runs a whorehouse." When I said Reinaldo seemed pleasant, David shook his head. "The kind of man I can't understand at all," he said. "His lover is a gringo, an older gentleman, a landscaper from Florida. He met Reinaldo when he was down here on a vacation, and when he retired he divorced his wife and left his home and his children and came to Mérida to be with Reinaldo. Who pays him back for such loyalty by cheating on him.

"Not me," David added. "I can only be with one man at a time."

A handsome fat man with a red beard was peering in the window of the store. We watched silently until he moved on.

"A Jew," David announced.

"How do you know?"

"I can always tell a Jew. It's easy."

The phone rang. David was being called home for *comida*. We went outside, he locked up, then got out a hook on a pole to grab the roll-down metal door that secures the front of his shop. I had thought he was through on the subject of his friend Reinaldo, but as we walked toward the corner, he said again, "Can you imagine? He has his gringo lover here and his Algerian lover in France and even that's not enough for him, so he brings the one from France back here and makes it into a three-way. How could anyone do that? Reinaldo doesn't think of anyone but himself."

I took David out to supper and over the meal in a mild, pleasant way he let me know I could sleep with him if I wanted to. When I first met David I found him attractive enough. But there was something abject about him, the heat in his stories was always about being cheated—by music publishers over his songs, in love by other men—and the question of why he'd never had success.

He was aware of it. Speaking of a man he called the love of his life, he said, "I know I am *something* of a masochist, but even so I couldn't take it the way it was going with this man. So eventually I broke it off. And for months—for years—I couldn't see him, couldn't pass him in the street without breaking down and crying." Later, over drinks at "Buffalo," a disco on the broad, fashionable avenue called the Montejo: "I have always lacked self-confidence. I have lived my life too much in fear. But now it's getting better for me."

We had gone to "Buffalo" because the owner owed David money on two necklaces he had purchased. He was supposed to be there by a particular hour, but he was very late even by the promiscuous standard invoked locally as "Mérida time." When he finally arrived, at first he claimed not to have the funds in the bank to cover the check. Then, while the owner was away talking on the phone, David pointed out to me that he was a Lebanese and, like all of them, always wanted to see if they could cheat you.

Bitter as he seemed about most things, David's stories of his own erotic life were sometimes very romantic. One was about meeting a man, younger than himself, married. His job was delivering tin goods to stores and to people's houses, and he was so attractive that when David would see him, he would throw up whatever he was doing and follow the guy through the streets just to get another glimpse of him. Finally, one day the younger man stopped David and confronted him, "What do you think you're doing?" he said. But he said it smiling, not in a mean way, so David took his life in his hands and said he couldn't do anything else, because he found the other man so attractive. And the guy said, "Well, do you want to do anything about it or do you just want to follow me around?" They went to a public bath, the one at the Hotel Colón, where they took a room. The rest of the younger man turned out to be as beautiful as his face was. And once they got started, it also turned out he was, as David put it, "*completamente masculino*," but also that he did everything—he fucked and could be fucked too. Eventually, he admitted he cared for David. He couldn't see him too often because of his marriage, but he would come around to the jewelry store, and David would close up and they'd go off someplace together. It lasted like that until the younger man had to move away to another city.

I met Joseph Gilbert one Saturday in March 1990, a heavyset, gray-bearded man in his fifties in a black *guayabera* and loose khaki pants.

Though he has since moved to Los Angeles, at the time Joseph had a small congregation of the gay and lesbian Metropolitan Community Church (MCC) in Philadelphia. He and his lover had traveled through the Yucatán one time on vacation and so, when his parishioners offered to pay for him to take a sabbatical for several months, Joseph came to Mérida and rented a house. Now his time was about up. Sunday night he was taking the bus across to Cancún, and then a flight home from there.

We were coming up the shady side of 62nd Street Sunday afternoon when Joseph asked me if I'd seen the baths at the Colón. I hadn't, I said, though I'd heard about them and the Colón was right across from where I was staying. So we went in the dark, cool lobby and Joseph asked could we be shown the Turkish baths. Did we want to *have* a bath? they asked. No, just to see them, we said.

An old attendant took us through. An inlaid plaque on the wall said the baths were built between 1942 and 1944 with state funds. Tile floors, marble or fake marble, art deco styling, all very deluxe and clean. We were taken into #7, one of the two more elegant and expensive suites, where there were cane rocking chairs, a steam room, a stone massage table, places to lie down and rest, and a small private swimming pool. As he understood it, Joseph said, the pools were refilled fresh for each new set of patrons.

"Are you having adventures here?" he asked.

"Well, I haven't been—," I said. "What about you?"

"Almost not," he said. "But if I were, I think one of these would be a good place to spend an hour getting to know someone."

I saw Joseph off on the 9:00 P.M. express for Cancún. Then, as I was walking back uptown from the bus station, under the mercury glow of the lamps in the park in front of the church of Santiago, I noticed a group of six or eight young men standing around among the parked cars. They were in their late teens and early twenties. As I came toward them, one of the bigger ones picked up one of the smaller ones, and the smaller one clamped his legs around the bigger one's hips. The bigger one made motions as though he were humping the smaller guy, and the smaller one was pretending he was enjoying the ride. The rest were all whistling and laughing at them.

I called and made an appointment to see Dr. Góngora again. His news this time concerned prostitutes and bisexual men. The female prostitutes he and his colleagues had been following in Mérida were not showing up with VIH infection at any meaningful rate. The only ones who were seropositive became so because of their (regular or casual) relationships with bisexual men. The data seemed to confirm that when bisexual men step outside their fixed heterosexual relationships, it is to have sex with other men. So the risk of becoming VIH-positive remained mostly among homosexual and bisexual men. "It turns out," Góngora said, "that women in Mérida do not have many sex partners outside their marriages. And in fact, neither do men."

Some of his own most productive education sessions, the doctor told me, had been when he went out to the Mayan towns. Because they were brought up around animals, the children there understood sex in a more biological and frank version than some young people in the city, he said.

He then introduced me to a younger doctor, Pedro González-Martínez, who had been his co-author in some of their studies and who had also been giving talks about SIDA in the Mérida schools. Pedro told me that his usual presentation is between forty-five minutes and an hour, never longer because after that the students start to lose attention. He began, he said, with an overview of the virus from a scientific point of view, then discussed methods of transmission. He encouraged the students to think about sexual contacts they may have had, even quite some time ago, and whether they might be at risk and should consider taking a "SIDA test." Then he allowed plenty of time for questions.

I asked Pedro if he handed out condoms or showed students how to use them. "No," he said. "Some people were doing that, and they ran into trouble. They came from Mexico City, and their real agenda was to promote—" Pedro looked at me. I was sure he was about to say "homosexuality." Instead, he said "—unusual practices."

Through Dr. Góngora I also met Judith Ortega Canto, a young physician connected with the Noguchi Center as a researcher in what is called social medicine. "Dr. Judy" is the author of a book, *Henequén y salud*, which is a meticulous study of living conditions among people on a henequén hacienda that has come into village collective ownership as an *ejido*. For well over a century sisal, the white fiber extracted from the spears of the giant henequén plant, was a major source for the world's twine and rope. At one point, Yucatán produced a third of the entire supply; "green gold," as henequén was called, made the state the wealthiest in Mexico. But in the 1960s the international market for sisal fell apart, largely because of the introduction of plastic substitutes in bailing procedures. At that point the owners were allowed to sell off their vast plantations to the government, which then turned most of them over to the workers. Dr. Judy's book tells a sad, complex story of increasing malnutrition and worsening health for people whose lives are saddled now to an agricultural industry that has gone bust. At the time Dr. Judy and I talked, she had moved on to a study of the attitudes of patients in the public psychiatric hospital toward the institution and toward their being incarcerated there. "On some level it's a very touching thing," she said, "these people looking for dignity, recognition of themselves as human beings."

I showed her an article from the previous day's paper about there being six men with VIH disease in the penitentiary in Mérida and no specialized treatment available to them. Did she believe that? Yes, Dr. Judy said, that would certainly make sense. The rejection of those with VIH or SIDA here was tremendous. Doctors, administrators, hospital workers—they all tried to avoid people who were infected. Married men were subject to *doble rechazo* (double rejection) by their wives, first for SIDA, then for what it revealed about their surreptitious sex life.

Well, then, who *was* actually taking care of people who had the disease?

Judy gave me the number of a woman who was working with something called the Association Against SIDA. Someone else was involved too, she said, at Social Security, a doctor named Guerrero, but she didn't have his phone number.

Dr. Góngora's statement that women in Mérida—and their husbands—do not have much sex outside marriage seemed to me wishful thinking. Against it, I could juxtapose the opinion of one gringo I had known, a long-time resident in Mérida married to a Yucatec woman, who had told me it was his impression that *all* married people in the city were having some sort of extramarital affair at all times. Strangely enough, a footnote in an older "scientific" source, Morris Steggerda's *Maya Indians of Yucatán* (1941), echoes the gringo's assertion:

> It is estimated that perhaps 50 percent of the Mayan men remain true to one woman throughout their entire lives. This percentage is higher than that for the Spanish-speaking classes, about whom I received four independent estimates from persons well qualified to form an opinion. One, a young man of 25 years, estimated that only 20 percent of Yucatecan men remained true to their wives. Another, an American having lived for many years in Yucatán, estimated that 1 or 2 percent remained true. The other two men, both past 60 years of age, were Yucatecans and said that in their opinion there were no Yucatecans who remained true to one woman throughout their entire lives.[2]

I remember Góngora-Biachi informing me the first time we met that epidemiology was not a subject their students could study at the University of Yucatán Medical School, as there were no epidemiologists on staff. His own training in diseases of the blood brought SIDA to him, and some of his conclusions make perfect sense as long as they are treated as lab results and are not held up to the test of actual human behavior. For example, he and his colleagues used several studies—by themselves and others—to come up with percentages of HIV-positive members of key groups. In stating the finding, however, they inadvertently use these figures to misinterpret their own information:

> For Mérida we have estimated that in 1990 the risk of acquiring VIH-1 infection through homosexual practices is from 15 to 20 percent, through sexual relations with prostitutes 0.5 percent and through transfusion 0.01 percent. The risk of acquiring VIH-1 in a population without risk practices is almost 0.[3]

This last would, of course, be not only true but also consoling *if* it turned out that the casual estimates of marital infidelity (especially of male bisexuality) in Mérida were wrong.

Their data about adolescent boys allow Góngora and his colleagues to posit that "a significant proportion of high school students in our city could be at risk of becoming infected through homosexual practices, even though these were casual." The writers understand that, at the moment, education is still the best prevention, but they believe the information should be controlled and dealt out differently to different sorts of people ("thus, for example, it is not the same thing to give information to a group of homosexuals as to a group of prostitutes"), and that the education of the general public "should be focused on avoiding risky sexual practices rather than on preventing infection through these types of practices."[4]

One of Mérida's cherished entertainment figures is an aging vaudeville clown named Héctor Herrera "Cholo." The lobby of the theater where "Yucatán's own" plays his loosely plotted shows is full of photos of him, many of them featuring Héctor in drag. "Cholo" is his major character, a cagey mestizo with sex eternally on his mind. Héctor's wife also stars in their revue, a sixty-ish woman who gets a laugh every time she sticks her big bosom in somebody's face or turns her big fanny to them. The show is a working-class, family event. Parents, grandparents and young children all attend. The joking runs to puns on words in Maya, which everyone in the audience except the lone gringo present finds hilarious. At one point a mestiza lady in a *huipil* is getting a guy on his knees all worked up by letting him rub her leg while she chats with somebody else. The guy on his knees gets so hot he starts also rubbing the leg of the man next to him. When the actors see what's going on, somebody comments, "*Pues, cuando se pica, se pica*," (Well, when you're bit, you're bit; or, When you're hot, you're hot).

Meridianos like to explain their "heat" or their sexiness or their preoccupation with sex as the result of their being Yucatecs or because they are hot-country, hot-blooded people or because they are Latins. (On the slight evidence of Héctor Herrera's little farces, it would appear Mayan people similarly would claim *their* sexiness as a *Mayan* trait.) The belief is variously self-forgiving, self-indulgent, self-aggrandizing, and self-castigating.

North of the border culture critics like to point out that one way the gay male movement of the last twenty-five years has affected the "mainstream" imagination has been to focus attention on the potential for sexual desirability of the male buttocks. For Latins, mainstream or not, this fact would hardly count as a "discovery." It was brought home to me quite strongly late one evening when Bill Ballantyne and I went to a club called La Cascada, where the clientele was young, mostly middle-class boys who came together in groups to get drunk and make connections with female prostitutes. As we were being shown to a table, up on the raised dance floor and bandstand a plump girl named Lidia was attaching a leather belt with maracas on it around the backside of a broadly built teenager. Before she would dance with him, Lidia made the blushing kid turn his butt to the audience and show them how well he could shake those maracas while the band drummer provided some rolls and rim shots and the crowd whistled and laughed and clapped.

Homosexual men in Mexico seem to accept without contention the idea that *their* heat or sexual appetite is large and barely under control. In a medical bookstore in the D.F. in 1989 I fell into conversation with a pleasant young clerk who assured me, "We Mexicans are very promiscuous, señor." When I mentioned that with SIDA the average period from infection to symptoms could be eleven years, this young man said, "Then what am I going to do? Not have sex with anybody?" and he laughed, as though we both understood the impossibility of *that*. Another time I was telling a gay medical doctor I know about the work on homosexuality of U.S. anthropologists Joe Carrier and Clark Taylor, and my friend remarked, "And what do they conclude? That we're even bigger *putos* than they are, right?"

On a holiday in honor of Benito Juárez, I was sitting on a bench in the park at Santa Lucia reading the *Diario* when Reinaldo Burgos, the man with the gringo lover I had met in David Muna's shop, came up to me. He'd been off buying gifts to take to people on his trip to France.

His lover was in the States, he said, returning this afternoon. They'd been together six years. They had a circle of friends they had cocktails with at least once a week, other English speakers, Reinaldo usually the only Mexican present. "And they all love me," he said.

His English was colloquial: "I'm no chicken hawk." "I gave him a blowjob." "I like my men masculine."

I asked if he knew what had happened to Los Charros, the little nightclub up the street with the funny round *travesti* M.C. I had been by there one night and it seemed to have gone out of business. Reinaldo said, "The police—or the government—started charging them too much in taxes and they closed it. The guy who owned it also owns all the whorehouses in town, but they still pushed him on this one."

I told Reinaldo I was having a hard time getting a handle on how people in Mérida felt about gays. Some of what I heard made the town appear very tolerant, some of it not.

"Oh basically they accept them," Reinaldo said. "The age for boys is the time before they get married, from about fifteen until they're twenty-four. They have their *novias*, their girlfriends, but the families are very careful about their girls, about protecting their virginity, so the boys also have a special friend, another boy they have sex with. Sometimes they give up the special friend when they get married and sometimes they don't. These are the ones who become bisexuals later on."

"And how do they decide who's going to be the *penetrator*?"

"They change off. It doesn't matter. They do it to each other, and when they get up from the bed one doesn't feel any less masculine than the other."

Then he told me two stories, mostly in English:

"One time, I was about twenty-six and I was in Monterrey in the north in this straight bar, and the waiter showed up with two beers that had been sent over to me. I asked him, 'What are these for? I don't know anyone here,' and the waiter just said they were from another table. Then after a while the men there waved me over, so I went. They were all four of them straight guys, talking about their baseball and about their adventures with prostitutes and then after a while I said I thought I was going to leave and the man who'd sent the beer squeezed my leg under the table and said why didn't I wait for him. He was about my age, and that was the first I knew for sure that something was going on. We walked back to my hotel and he said he had a bottle in his car and why didn't he come up and we'd drink it, so we did. He said he fucked his wife and he went with prostitutes but when he was with another man he liked to get fucked, so I did it to him and he kept saying, 'That's good, that's good, give it to me.' "

The other story: "One night a few years ago, it was about eleven o'clock, I was sitting in the park across from the Café Express and a man in his forties came up and asked me if I was gay. I told him well—I didn't really say anything, so then he said he was married and had children and he lived in Michigan and in his fantasies he had thought about other men but he'd never done anything about it. Then he asked me if I'd like to come up to his hotel room and I went. He didn't know how to do anything with another man and he was very afraid, his hands were trembling. He didn't even know how to take another man's clothes off him, and I started to show him and he shot off in his pants. Then he started apologizing over and over and I told him not to worry, and I undressed him and we got on the bed and I played with him and he played with me. I gave him a blowjob and he gave me one, and then we spent the night making love. In the morning he kissed me and said, 'I'll always remember you.' "

Before he went home to get things straightened up for the return of "Fred" from the States, Reinaldo said, "I've had sex with a certain number of women in my life, five maybe, and they always ask me how it is I know how to do certain things—to pull out before I have my orgasm, or let them have theirs first—and I tell them it's because I'm gay and gays know how to give pleasure to others, that I've practiced it. And they say, well from now on they're going to look for gay men to have sex with. Straight men, all they know is how to get their own pleasure. A lot of them, ten minutes and they're done."

I went back to have coffee with Eddie at his desk upstairs at the famous curio shop. He was walking with a slight limp, but he told me he was well. I thanked him for the leads he had given me before, said I had learned something about SIDA since then.

"Have you?" he said.

Then, a scant minute later, he was back to his old song: "Me, I don't give a shit. I had my share and now I don't have any and if they ever find a vaccine for it I'll be too old. A rifle left unused *rots*, you know. I don't even say anything to my nephews. I don't give a shit. They can read. These old faggots who live here all have their sixteen-year-old boys and if I say to *them*, 'Take care of yourself,' you know what they say? 'Why? This guy's paying me 20,000 pesos every time I do it with him.' "

And in the villages? Did he think it was true the boys there began with men, or with other boys?

"Of course. What else can they do? They can't have the girls, so when they get an erection they go and do it to each other. Or some older guy comes along. Then they're fifteen and they get a girl pregnant and they get married, and if he doesn't like her they separate and he finds another girl. What do I care what they do to each other? It's their life. The kids who work for me, I don't care what they do either, as long as they don't do it in the back of my place. If their little girlfriends call here more than twice in one week asking for them, I say, 'He doesn't work here anymore.' And if they ask why, I say, 'Because I just fired him.' I've never once had anything sexual to do with any of my workers in any of my businesses. I made it my rule.

"And don't think they care at the national level either. If they did, they would have done something by now. Or up north where you come from either. All those millions of dollars they put out for research . . . where are they? That guy in your country, it didn't save him."

"Who?"

"That designer. Halston. He died this morning. It was on the radio.

"I cut my own hair these days, you know. I'm afraid of getting a prick at the barber's. And I keep a bottle of alcohol there on the shelf and after I clip my nails I wash the clippers before I put them back in the drawer. You don't know. My sister's husband uses the same clippers. Who knows where he goes at night? None of my business anyway, and certainly not something I want to have to think about!"

In the Shade of the Ya'ax Che

MARCH 1990–SEPTEMBER 1992

It was Joseph Gilbert, the MCC minister, who introduced me to a seventy-page book called *Nuevos enfoques sobre la homosexualidad* (New approaches to homosexuality), written by a priest in Mérida, Ricardo Zimbrón Levy. A surprising, positive, enlightened piece of work, Joseph said. After reading as much of it as he could with his limited Spanish, he had gone to hear Father Ricardo's Sunday mass. Afterward, when Joseph went up and introduced himself, Father Ricardo had invited him to come again and co-celebrate with him. Though Joseph hadn't thought that the right thing for him to do, the offer had pleased him a great deal.

Father Zimbrón belongs to the Missionaries of the Holy Spirit, a Mexican order that has a church they call "Nuestra Señora de la Consolación," located a block off the Zócalo. Originally a convent of another order, the place is better known in Mérida as "Las Monjas." On the corner, in front of the chapel and the main temple, is a walled-in patio shaded by large trees. Inside the huge stone church most of the decoration has been removed. Above the altar hangs a big wooden cross and a giant, oval, unframed painting of Our Lady in Her grief. The Sunday morning I went with Joseph, an earlier mass was just ending. Crowds streamed from the church, jostling the people waiting to get in. The congregation was made up of poorer people from the center of town, more women than men, everyone freshly bathed and powdered and lightly scented, the men with their hair slicked back. There was a newsprint handout with the responses and the day's lessons for them to follow. Father Ricardo turned out to be a balding man of about sixty with a light, almost faint voice, even when he spoke directly into the microphone beside him. Instead of a heavy sermon, he gave a reasonable, plain talk mainly about how Jesus expects us to judge things in terms of our own conscience. The music for the service most of the congregation knew by heart. They sang along to the earnest strumming of a guitar, the echoing rising over the hum of the electric fans stationed around the church. Hundreds of people lined up to go forward and receive the Host and I thought we would be there forever, but everyone moved right along, up to the railing, back to the pews, and the service was over in forty minutes.

Father Ricardo's *New Approaches to Homosexuality* begins, "I am an old priest who daily, for more than thirty years, has heard the confession of many people." In all that time, the priest says, he has encountered many people who want to rid themselves of their homosexuality. They try over and over, with all their might and main, but usually without much success. Then two things happen: the penitent stops coming to confession and the confessor is left frustrated, aware that he has done no good and probably has even contributed to the penitent's sense of his own impotence in the face of this problem. As a result, Father Ricardo admits, he has begun to doubt the wisdom of the Church on the subject, restated most recently in the 1986 pastoral letter of Romanian cardinal Joseph Ratzinger, Prefect of the Congregation for the Doctrine of the Faith. Is "absolute chastity or mortal sin" a possible set of alternatives for ordinary people? Zimbrón doesn't think so. He quotes both Jesus in Matthew and Saint Paul in Corinthians as acknowledging that the gift or vocation for sexual abstinence is given to very few. The Vatican's position not only conflicts with the findings of modern biological and social science, Father Zimbrón says, for a pastoral counselor like himself it also creates a crisis of conscience. By writing the book, which is dedicated to other priests and educators, to parents and to homosexuals, he says he feels he is "paying a debt to a good percentage of Christ's flock for whom nothing has been done, except perhaps for making their situation worse."

For his research, Father Zimbrón has read eclectically: Freud, Kinsey, Wilhelm Reich, Dennis Altman, Joe Carrier, current Catholic liberal moralists like the Spanish Reverend Father Marciano Vidal, even Will Durant on ancient Greece and the homophobic members of the psychiatric establishment of the 1950s and 1960s like Irving Bieber. Sorting the possible "causes" of homosexuality, he weighs theories that many gays and lesbians in the United States would want to dismiss as out of date, such as the question of whether an adolescent may become gay through "social contagion" or pressure from adult homosexuals and milieu, as well as theories like "genetic predisposition" whose fortunes continue to rise and fall.

Whatever the antecedents of homosexual longings, Zimbrón recognizes them as being, above all, part of creation and not in themselves sinful. The only "sin" he sees stemming from homosexuality is the sin of parents rejecting their own children. The form the rejection will generally take depends on the family's economic condition, according to Zimbrón. Where the homosexual direction of a son is recognized early, the working-class father (himself "almost always a machista") will usually shun the boy completely or subject him to ridicule and verbal abuse, while the mother is more likely to suffer through, trying to make the best of the situation. She may not reject her son, "but neither will she welcome him with open arms or take much pride in him."[5] On the other hand, the middle- or upper-class family's main preoccupation will be with the "social image of the family" and the "social disgrace implicit in having a member of the family be homosexual." The implication is that the working-class family does not have the resource to attempt to control the image it presents the world, while the middle- or upper-class family either does or at least supposes it does.

Father Ricardo assures mothers and fathers of all classes of the complete uselessness of trucking a child with homosexual tendencies about to doctors, psychiatrists, or priests to get him "fixed." What he says is needed—and often completely lacking, especially in Mexico—is understanding on the part of the family. The child who receives care and acknowledgement "feels worthy, he perceives himself as a person of dignity because he is loved."

After I had read the *Nuevos enfoques*, I went back to Las Monjas on a weekday morning and attended Father Ricardo's mass again. Afterward, members of the congregation waited for him in the sunny interior courtyard between the church and the residence and the classrooms. Once he had taken off his vestments, Father Ricardo came padding out in jeans and sandals, no socks, a T-shirt, and a striped short-sleeve shirt with the tails hanging out. Some had short questions to ask, others little personal contributions they wanted to put into his hand. When my turn came, I told Father Ricardo who I was, mentioned Father Joseph Gilbert, and asked if I could talk with him a moment. "Of course," he said, "just wait for me." When the others were finished, he showed me into a living room with high-back Victorian-style furniture upholstered in shiny red, offered me a chair, and sat next to me on a sofa.

I said I had heard that a lot of homosexuals were in his congregation, including people with SIDA. Yes, Father Ricardo said, that was true. Was that why he had written the book? In part, yes. Another reason was that his own brother had had a homosexual son, and both parents—Father Ricardo's brother and his sister-in-law—had treated the boy with a good deal of understanding and his life had turned out well for him.

"Mexico, you know," Father Ricardo said, "is a country where, unfortunately, there is a great failure of learning—of education—among the middle and lower classes. So when problems like this come up, people don't have access to the latest information, and they fall back on traditional ways of doing things and thinking about things." He stopped himself and laughed. "Though, at least we don't have the problem of being founded by the Puritans that you have up there. Do *you* understand the Puritans? The Fundamentalists? So full of hatred."

No, I said, I didn't understand them at all.

The evils of *rechazo* (rejection) are a major theme of the *Nuevos enfoques*. When the young person who has been ridiculed by his peers and shunned by his own parents goes to his parish priest for help, Father Ricardo writes, he discovers that, according to the Catholic Church, God also rejects him. Under such pressure, an adolescent may lose all sense of himself as a thing of value. Rejected by others, he will eventually begin to loathe himself. No one can be expected to withstand the opinion of the world forever, says Father Ricardo. If we are told over and over that we are worthless—"trash"—then that is how we will begin to act.

"The most important lesson in that book," Father Ricardo told me, "is the idea that nobody else can enter within the boundaries of your own conscience. Not Father Ratzinger or any of the fathers of the Church. Nobody. What my conscience says to me is the most important thing."

With practice, he writes, we ourselves can learn what it is God wants of us. In the silence of prayer we will begin to hear Him. (The role Father Ricardo sees for a pastoral guide like himself is only to show the paths available, never to prescribe, castigate, or condemn.) We are wholly "knowable" as individuals (God at least knows us), which means our desires and the arrangement of our sexual lives are *not* somehow different from the rest of our business. Here, too, God is trying to help us know ourselves. Father Ricardo stresses the conclusion that our earthly love for one another, including but not confined to erotic love, is part and parcel of our highest humanity and our most profound spirituality. Ironically, at times he achieves a tone very much like that of Saint Paul, who so abhorred everything sexual:

> Now love which is faithful and constant is a very high virtue, truly beneficial and hard to sustain, because it implies the renunciation of all egoism, and requires a large measure of self denial, disinterest and sacrifice in honor of the person we love. Anyone capable of living in true love I would give a "10" in morals. This I learned from the Gospel.[6]

Wise as Father Ricardo is, at times he does not seem to understand how messy the entanglements of secular life can be. "We can affirm, without doubt," he says, "that true love implies a good dose of prudence and sanity. A sexual relation which brings on situations that are embarrassing for one person, or for the couple, cannot be an authentic act of love."

In the book, he quotes a gay Canadian journalist talking about the tremendous pain of his own disillusionment with the Church. I found myself telling Father Ricardo about Ray. "I have lived almost thirteen years with the same man. He was born Catholic, but because of his sexuality since adolescence he has felt rejected or at least badly understood by his own church. Now he has HIV, although he is still without symptoms, and faces all this without believing he has any spiritual resources for the fight to come."

"Oh no, that's wrong," said Father Ricardo. "Tell him none of us is lacking in those. Tell him we here will be praying for him."

I was about to leave when I remembered that in the *Enfoques* Father Ricardo had spoken about one kind of homosexuality as being based on a "purely" biological situation. I asked if he knew examples of that. Father Ricardo said, "One young man came to see me simply to ask if I knew where in Mexico he could get a sex-change operation. He works here in town. His chest is very well developed and he wears loose shirts to hide his breasts. The penis isn't so well developed and he does have a womb. The doctors say he might even be able to have children in the long run. Do you know where they do these operations? In Tijuana? Where?"

I said I didn't know the answer to that one either, but I would ask around.

And then, outside in the sun, Father Ricardo said, "If you've been together so long in a couple, how did your friend contract the virus?"

"There's a long period from infection to the onset of symptoms," I said. "They now think it's an *average* of eleven years."

"Ah—," he said, nodding, smiling.

I went away glad that I had had the courage to go in and meet him, and sorry that I hadn't been able to confess to him that the reason we think Ray is HIV-positive and I am not is because our relationship has never been completely monogamous.

Something—perhaps their enormous sense of what it means to be civil, or the desire to keep me from seeing their city in a bad light—kept people I talked with about SIDA in 1988 and 1990 from mentioning the days of the moral campaign against homosexuals in May 1987. I learned about the incident instead from clips from national newspapers put together by Max Mejía, an activist, editor, and translator, in an excellent collage chronicle of public response to the epidemic in Mexico called *SIDA: Historias extraordinarias del siglo XX* (AIDS: Strange stories of the twentieth century):

> Mérida, Yucatán
> Under the slogan "may God help us in this campaign" a "witchhunt" has been initiated against homosexuals, lesbians and transvestites, which has as its goal the eradication of "immoral sex practices" and an end to the spread of SIDA (Síndrome de Inmunodeficiencia Adquirida). In an action that recalls the medieval crusades, parent associations, university student groups, and Catholic groups, some sponsored by private initiative, seek to have "homosexuals and lesbians denounced publicly, as they are the ones who have brought on SIDA." This morning, all the schools and faculties of the Universidad Autónoma de Yucatán awoke to find themselves inundated with broadsides and posters urging children and young people to denounce homosexual attitudes and calling for judicial action against them. They also urge the closing of nightclubs "where transvestite homosexuals and bisexuals work." The posters all agree on the necessity of public exposure of homosexuals and those who live with them. Some of the advertisements proclaim in large type, "Denounce homosexuals and lesbians," and then explain the need to eliminate such people from the parks and public places they frequent. The justification given is that SIDA has spread in Yucatán because of homosexuals, and this is the reason legal action against them is sought. The posters and slogans are signed by the Union of Padres de Familia of Mérida, Catholic University Youth, Youth and Promise, and Youth, Love, and Strength, among other groups, which are sponsored by the organization that goes under the name of the National Association for Morality, headed by Yucatec business leader Victor Arjona Barbosa.
>
> (Roberto Fuentes Vivar, *La Jornada*, May 4, 1987)

"However," as Max Mejía writes, "the siege does not prosper. Doctors and civil society stave it off at once; they confront it and denounce it for what it is: a piece of political blackmail from the right.

"The opinion of the head of health services in Yucatán, Dr. Oscar Cuevas Graniel, the same day as the actions:

> There is no crime to prosecute against homosexuals. They have begun to take the health measures needed against the spread of SIDA, just as strict controls over blood transfusions have been instigated.
>
> (Roberto Fuentes Vivar, *La Jornada*, May 7, 1987)

"Dr. Alejandro Guerrero, specialist in infectious and contagious diseases at the IMSS in Mérida:

> We must stop satanizing people with SIDA and homosexuals. It is as though we were still in the era when the leper had a bell put on him and was left alone to die, like an untouchable!
>
> (*La Jornada*, May 8, 1987)

"Dr. Victor Torrás, specialist in hematology at the Hospital Centro Médico of IMSS:

> A hunt against homosexuals has been undertaken, distorting the information we have about the disease. SIDA is being used against homosexuals, even though they aren't responsible either for the appearance of the illness or for its spread.
>
> (*La Jornada*, May 20, 1987)

"The official spokesman of the archbishopric of Mérida assures us that they do not know of the existence of the organizations Youth, Love, and Strength, Youth and Promise, or Yucatec Catholic Youth." (Ibid.)

In lowland Maya the *ya'ax che* is the ceiba, or silk cotton tree. Native to the peninsula the ceiba reaches impressive size and spread, and at one season of the year produces bolls of white fluff at the ends of its branches. Harvested, the fluff becomes kapok, which is used as stuffing in furniture and cheap sleeping bags like the ones we took on Boy Scout overnights when I was a kid. For the people of the time before the Conquest, the shade of the *ya'ax che* provided the image for tranquility after struggle, Heaven as they conceived it. According to Bishop Landa, the Maya, like us, imagined two quite different places for human souls to spend eternity:

> The evil life of suffering they say was for the vicious, and the good and delectable for those whose mode of life had been good. The delights they said they would come into if they had been of good conduct, were by entering a place where nothing would give pain, where there would be abundance of food and delicious drinks, and a refreshing and shady tree they called *Yaxche'* [Landa's orthogra-

phy], the Ceiba tree, beneath whose branches and shade they might rest and be in peace forever.

The *ya'ax che* has also been appropriated as the name and logo for Mérida's small, volunteer SIDA organization, where the tree is sometimes pictured as an umbrella giving protection against the rain. "Ya'ax Che, the Association Against SIDA in the Southeast" was begun in September 1989 in response to the feeling of a small number of people that none of the governmental organizations—city, state, or federal—were paying enough attention to education about safe sex, to the anti-homosexual educational campaigns of the Right, or to the desperate need in which some of the people who had contracted SIDA found themselves. A house downtown a block and a half from Santa Lucia Park was rented to serve as an office and almost at once a young man named José Luis Matú, who had been drummed out of the place he lived when his neighbors discovered he was VIH-positive, moved into the back rooms. Alejandro Guerrero was the Association's first president. Lizbet Castilla, who owns POP, the coffee shop across from the university, and the restaurant El Patio del Peregrino next door, became the group's treasurer. A brusque, good-looking, efficient woman, "Liz" (pronounced "Leese") worked as a medical secretary before getting started in the restaurant business. From the beginning, there were serious difficulties for Ya'ax Che as a charity, Liz told me. For one thing, the Association failed to become "fashionable." "People will give money to homes for old people, but they don't want to get connected—or get their names associated—with this SIDA business in any way," she said. Support that might be expected from the families of those with the disease was also not forthcoming. Alejandro pointed out to me once that mothers often expect that once their sons know they have SIDA they will "give up all this homosexuality." "But then their sons don't change," he said, "and the mothers would come to a couple of meetings at the Association and see the transvestites and some of the gayer people, and it would make them uncomfortable and they'd not come back another time."

At the end of 1989 the Association gave some safe-sex workshops in schools, and a month later there was a complaint, a letter from an engineer who belonged to the *Pro Vida* movement, published in the *Diario de Yucatán*. The engineer said that Jaime Sepulveda Amor, director of CONASIDA, the government SIDA office in the D.F., had been denounced for publicizing the use of *preservativos* (condoms) and stopped from doing it, and now the same business had reared its head "in our own Yucatán." Alejandro or one of the other members would always dutifully write a response to such letters because the *Diario* is so influential in the peninsula. But they never felt they were winning the battle that way. When I asked Alejandro if he and some other doctors couldn't prevail on the *Diario* to change its policy, he sighed. "They'd say, 'Oh we'll print what you write,' but then for every letter or article that was pro condom, they'd continue to run five against them."

That was 1990. Two years later when I come by to talk with Georgina Martínez González, the young woman who has become director, I get the sense that the Association continues to feel heavily beleaguered. Georgina has an office of her own in a room that can be closed off and locked. The fax machine is kept there, and the walls are decorated with the more explicit safe-sex posters, all of which come from the United States (the one I notice is from the San Francisco AIDS Foundation, a black and white photograph of a seated young man with the erect penis covered by a condom and the slogan "Dress for the Occasion"). In one corner is the sex-lecture equipment, including boxes of condoms and a big pink dildo; in another, shelves of medical supplies and cans of nutritional supplement for people who can't afford to buy them.

Georgina works in sales in the morning, then comes in to volunteer her time at the Ya'ax Che office from 4:00 P.M. until 8:00 or 9:00 at night. She takes out Marlboros and offers me one. When I refuse, she apologizes for her habit, asks me if I mind if she goes ahead. She came here from Ciudad Carmen in Campeche to get a medical degree, but she had to work to put herself through school, and toward the end she just got *tired* of the whole thing and didn't finish. Now she gives most of the *charlas* (talks) about safe sex that the Association is asked to put on. I recall Alejandro telling me before they had had some success using medical students to give these talks. "Yes," Georgina says, "but often the students have complicated schedules and can't come at the appointed time, and since my time is more easily rearranged, I've begun doing the majority of them."

She wishes she didn't feel forced into doing all the ordinary work of the office. "If only we had someone we could pay to be here and answer the phone. There *are* other volunteers, but their schedules change all the time and—" Georgina would like to pursue SIDA and safe-sex education for women, prostitutes especially. I mention the article I saw in the *Diario* two years ago claiming there were six cases of SIDA in the local penitentiary. "We've known about that," Georgina says. "We've wanted to have a prison education project, but I don't know how we could even begin that, who we could talk to." She turns to the problem of the homeless children begging in the streets. That's a terrible thing, the parents sending them out on the streets like that, making beggars of them. *Pandilleros* they're called. The city feeds them and allows them to stay over at the Casa del Pueblo on 65th Street, she says, but they don't actually *do* anything that would begin to eliminate the problem itself.

People here just don't care about things, Georgina says. The government *certainly* doesn't care. CONASIDA? It seems to have plenty of money to spend in the D.F., but does any of it ever get out and come to organizations in the other states like the Association? If so, Ya'ax Che hasn't seen any of it. The politicians? None of them has done anything about SIDA. The mayor of Mérida is a woman who belongs to the conservative party, the Partido Acción Nacional (PAN). The governor of the state, Dulci Maria Sauri, is a trained sociologist and the first woman to hold that office. But Dulci Maria is of the ruling PRI (Partido Revolucionario Institucional), so, as Georgina sees it, the two of *them* spend all their time and effort trying to embarrass each other.

It is the conservatism of Mérida that finally gets to her, Georgina says. "A slave mentality. They treat the Mayas as slaves, but the people of the city are also slaves themselves, slaves to their own pretensions. Anything 'new' or anything that comes from 'abroad'—they'll pay any amount for those things, purely as status symbols."

I am asking about the availability of the VIH test to people who aren't in the IMSS system when in comes José Luis Matú, the young man who lives in the back of the house. He has on Spandex shorts and a loose black undershirt, bracelets, necklaces, lots of silver rings, and a black porkpie hat with lavender glass triangles. "Matú" as he is called by everyone, has with him a cardboard box full of medications—including two bottles of AZT—which have been donated by the father of a young man who died last week. "He told me he didn't know exactly what all these things were for, but he hoped someone else could use them," Matú says.

Matú leaves. Georgina takes out a new cigarette. "At the O'Horán," she says, "where the people with no money go, the test for VIH costs 70,000 pesos (U.S. $23). So who would be able to take it there of their own free will?"

But I've read in their literature that CONASIDA promises sixty-eight locations in the country where you can get the VIH test for free.

"That's right. But *here*, in 'our Yucatán,' Salud Publica made the decision to charge everybody 70,000 pesos for it!"

I mention that on previous trips I had talks with Dr. Góngora-Biachi. "Góngora?" Georgina says. "Do you know what he did? Told the newspaper condoms don't work. Part of a plot by the homosexuals, he said. Well, he's gone out of SIDA work anyway. Got a big grant to study something involving blood from the Japanese."

In Georgina's time in medical school, all interns had to learn how to do proctology exams and check men's prostate glands. This was at the O'Horán Hospital. "There would be a male doctor present, the professor," she recalls, "but most of the patients were Mayan. To have to take down their pants and have a woman do that to them—the men would look like they were going to die of embarrassment."

One of the volunteers at the Association is a woman named Margot (pronounced Mar-GOT), seventy-six years old now, squat, gray-haired, wearing a dirty white nurse's or housekeeper's uniform. She has bright black eyes, tiny diamond earrings, a sweaty but not at all unpleasant smell. Margot has a bad heart, she tells me, and has to lose weight, so she's on a diet of almost nothing but fruit and vegetables. (Talking about her health, she slips her hand inside the collar of her uniform and touches her chest.) She is a widow. Her husband brought her to Mexico from Spain when she was seventeen or eighteen. He worked for Lázaro Cárdenas, the president of the Republic from 1934 to 1940 whose most famous deed was the nationalization of the Mexican oil industry. Cárdenas's son Cuauhtémoc ran as the liberal-reform Partido de la Revolución Democrática (PRD) candidate for the presidency in 1988 and, many believe, got a plurality of the popular vote.

"So you knew President Cárdenas?"

"Oh yes," says Margot.

"So you must know Cuauhtémoc too."

"When he was a boy I did," Margot nods. "But Cuauhtémoc is another matter entirely." She laughs and looks away, giving a dismissive little wave of her hand.

Margot and her husband lived in Mexico City. She had her children there, two boys. Then the earthquake of 1985 came and, though they were together the moment it happened, her husband was killed and Margot survived. "Forty years together," she says, "and then—. He died instantly." Afterward, Margot didn't have anything to do, so she came to Mérida where her sons are, and her grandchildren. She lives alone and volunteers her time, at the Red Cross and here at the Association.

"There is so much to do," she says. "I get up very early every morning and I eat a piece of fruit and have my shower, and then I'm ready and I go directly to the Red Cross. My job there is to make the connections that people need. The Red Cross, you know, is a rescue service. They can't keep people. The police call and our men go out in the middle of the night to the streets and it's a poor alcoholic who's fallen down and can't get up. Well, then in the morning when he comes around, I go in to him and I say, 'What do you want? Do you think if I could get you into a clinic you could get over this disease?' And sometimes they'll say, 'No, señora, don't waste your time. Once the treatment's over I'll just go and get drunk again as soon as I can get the money together to do it, you know.' But I tell them, 'No, I can't just leave you like this.' Especially the elderly, their families have thrown them out, or neglected them, they really don't know very well where they are anymore, and there aren't many places to send them. The old people's homes, maybe. But we do what we can. They're raising the funds now, maybe the Red Cross can have a facility of its own. Then in the afternoon when my work there is finished, I come here and do what I can. *These* poor people—this is an awful thing, too, and no one's doing anything about *it* either."

On a Sunday I come by the Association to get José Luis Matú and we walk up to the park at Santa Lucia, then down Calle 60, closed to traffic for Sunday strollers, toward the Zócalo. Dressed as usual in his Speedos, felt hat, and plenty of jewelry, Matú elicits from passersby stares, laughter, surprise—and also many hellos and waves from people he knows. As though he can read my mind, he says, "You know, they don't reject me, Charlie."

Three years ago, however, he came home one day to find the neighbor ladies rummaging through his place. "Señoras," he told them, "please! What do you think you're doing here? This is *my* house!" The neighbors had discovered his VIH status from their local doctor, and now they wanted all the little boys in the neighborhood to be forced to take the SIDA test. "And if any of *them* had come up positive," says Matú, "can you imagine what they would have done to *me*?"

We stop for lunch at the Bougainvillea, the coffee shop of the Hotel Balam, which is nearly empty. At first Matú says he won't have anything, just coffee, but then he changes his mind and has the aged waiter bring him a large order of french fries. Matú has lived in the States, and we talk back and forth between Spanish and his excellent English. Like Russell Rodriguez at the T-1, Matú has determined that the way to deal with the name "Carter" having no Spanish equivalent is to call me "Charlie."

Matú is thirty-two now. He has told me his first employment was as a desk clerk at the Mayaland and the Hacienda, the two tourist hotels at Chichén Itzá. So I ask if he knows anything much about the sexual lives of the Mayan men who worked either at the hotels or in the surrounding towns. Sorry, he says, but he doesn't. He was only seventeen or so and he was doing it with all kinds of guests at the hotel—for fun, for the fascination of it, not for money or getting ahead in business or anything—but he wasn't having anything to do with the rest of the staff.

Perhaps noticing my mild disappointment, Matú hurries on. His gay life began in earnest when he was seven, fucking for pleasure with a fourteen year old. (At the age of three he was held down and fucked by five year olds, but that *wasn't* pleasant.) He's still friends with that first guy. "He got married when he was in his twenties. 'To avoid trouble,' he told me. But he continues to see other men for sex and says to me he thinks he always will."

Matú left home when he was sixteen because of fights with his parents, worked in public relations in tourism, then moved to Los Angeles, where among other things he helped set up a latino arts organization called the Taller Frida Kahlo.

He pretends not to comprehend the politics of SIDA very well. "I need to study more," he says. But, perhaps from his career in public relations, he clearly does understand that one way to precipitate action is to cause as much embarrassment as you can. "I'm going to Miami," he says, "and I'm not going to any old governmental agency or anything, I'm going directly to the Catholic Church and I'm going to say, 'There are people where I come from over there in Yucatán who are dying from lack of nutrition. We need peanuts, we need *et cetera*.' That should get things started, don't you think, Charlie?"

He wants me to write a letter to the governor about kids selling Chiclets in the street and about the noise and about the hideous smoke of the trucks and how ugly it is, and how destructive to tourism. Just to embarrass her.

I say, "Let me stay a while in a subterranean role here."

"You mean in the closet?"

"No. Just let me do my work for a while before I have to make a stink with the governor."

Matú says OK, he'll write the letter himself.

He found out his father had made a will leaving half his house to Matú's brother and half to one of his sisters. So when he was there visiting, Matú said to his father, "I think I know why, but I want to hear it from your own mouth. Why aren't you willing a third part of the house to me?" His father said because then maybe Matú's older sister wouldn't want to live there. Then he said, "Or what if I were still alive and you brought one of your friends who's sick and they gave me SIDA?" (His father doesn't seem to understand that Matú is VIH-positive himself.)

Was he his mother's favorite, then? Did *she* care for him?

"My mother? She was, if possible, worse. In her old age she came to me and said, 'Now I'm sick and you'll have to take care of me.' But I said, 'Wait a minute *honey*. Let's look at this. Why should *I* take care of *you*? From the time I was ten years old you never paid for anything for me. Isn't that right? I earned the money myself. My sisters and my brother, you paid for their schooling. But me? Nothing. So why should I take care of you now?' " And Matú's mother, who has since died, said, "You're right, José Luis, you're right."

His sisters and his brother hate him going on television to talk about SIDA. " 'Why do you have to do that?' they say. 'Announce to the world that you're homosexual?' And I tell them," Matú says, 'Because that's what I am!' "

Alejandro Guerrero says that both at the T-1 and at the Association they receive criticism for allowing Matú to be a spokesman for them. Alejandro and Matú went on a television program one time with someone from Public Health, and afterward the public health official said to Alejandro, "Please, next time, don't bring someone like *that* around."

If you go to a professional conference and you bring someone who isn't your wife (a secretary, say), the *grosería* (foul thing) people may comment with is, "Oh, I see you brought along your *culo* (piece of ass)." Alejandro even gets that from his colleagues about José Manuel. One director of a hospital warned him not to take José Manuel to a conference in Cancún. "It makes you look bad," he said. Alejandro told him, "But it's an event where José Manuel has to make presentations. He's my assistant. You take *your* assistants along to conferences."

> *A Mexican worker earning the minimum salary in 1980 brought home the equivalent of U.S. $7.02 per day. By 1990 the minimum daily wage had fallen to U.S. $3.13.*[7]

That the standard of living has declined absolutely for half the people in Mexico in the last decade does not usually figure in the picture visitors get of Mexico in the current moment. But the people at Ya'ax Che and at the SIDA clinic at the IMSS T-1 Hospital—Matú, Margot, Alejandro, Georgina, José Manuel—continuously face certain effects of a declining economy in a country where half the people didn't have a formal "job" *before* the slide began: the children sent out to beg, the traffic in drugs, the fact that people with SIDA need not only expensive medications, but also to eat better, which many of them can't afford to do. These are some of what my friend John Borrego calls the "carefully hidden pains" that come from the bleeding of a nation by international capital.

People who live in Mérida, even those involved in the tourist industry, come not to notice tourists. In the POP or the Café Express, you can watch Meridianos sort with their eyes. Their gaze will jump over the latest lanky young blond couple with their backpacks and their mosquito bites and their guidebooks, here for three days, four at the most. The stories of suffering, including the SIDA stories, unfold in a universe parallel to and contiguous to the one the tourists inhabit. And though the two universes touch and touch again, they appear not to. I go walking downtown, and half the people I know to say hello to on the street are likely to be VIH-positive. But when the school teachers from Kansas City I meet by the pool at the Hotel Panamericana ask me what I'm doing here, and I say, "Some work on AIDS," and they say, "Oh, and is there AIDS here too?" their faces also register disappointment, as if to say, "What an unpleasant man to bring this up. Doesn't he know we're on vacation?"

Two years ago when I first talked with the songwriter and shopkeeper David Muna, he didn't know anyone personally who was infected with VIH. But now, he tells me this tale:

He had a vase, a fine thing he wanted made over into a lamp for his mother. He took it to the craftsman who he knew would do the best job, and there in the shop he caught sight of one of the most beautiful boys he had ever seen in his life. And it turned out when the lamp was finished it was that boy who was sent to deliver it. David then made the mistake of saying he loved the way the whole piece had been put together, but hated the shade. Too fussy, too ordinary, something—. The kid seemed put off by that, which meant to David that *he* must have been the one who made the shade. Then later, David found out that the craftsman who had done the lamp for him had SIDA, and that he had died. After that, David didn't come across the beautiful boy for a long time, and when he did, he could tell that he also had the disease. Completely ruined, none of his former beauty left. This boy had a brother, even more good looking if that was possible, and one day David ran into him. When David asked, the boy said, "My brother died." Then he told him, "Our maestro infected my brother, and then he infected me. I'm sick with it too."

I was downtown with Alejandro one afternoon when we passed David on the sidewalk. I introduced the two men and they shook hands. A few days later when I went by David's shop to invite him to come eat with me, a young man was visiting, leaning against the counter talking with David. This one, whose name I don't recall, spoke English, French, and German, David told me.

After a few minutes, David said, "I should warn you, Carter."

"About what?"

"Your new friend Guerrero. He is considered somewhat problematic around here."

"What does that mean?"

" 'Problematic,' as I said. I have friends who have had to leave the Association because of him."

I pressed a little, but David wouldn't say any more. I began to think the invitation to go to supper was a bad idea, so I don't issue one. But I stayed on a little while. We were talking about how much things are changing in the city and I said something about how even someone like David here, "*la dama de Mérida*"— (no excuse for my saying it), and David got angry. "What's this talk about *damas*?" he demanded. "I don't like it at all. I'm a man with a twenty-inch penis and an ass as good-looking as yours. *Et cetera*."

I apologized and soon after left the shop. I spoke to Alejandro, who said he and David had had words on a bus one day. A young man and woman got on and there were seats on either side of David, but he wouldn't move to let the couple sit together. Alejandro said something to him about it, but David still wouldn't move. Then another time on the street, David was behind Alejandro, and Alejandro set off running to catch a bus and David stepped on the back of his shoe.

I have another friend, Jorge Solís, a trained architect now in his thirties who works part-time at the Asociación Ya'ax Che. Jorge's original goal was to become a priest. At the age of twenty he went off to the D.F. to the seminary of the Missionaries of the Holy Spirit, Father Ricardo Zimbrón's order. But it turned out that other priests in the Misioneros were not, as Jorge puts it, as "advanced" in their thinking about certain things as Father Ricardo is. At the time Jorge was not troubled about the possibility of his being a homosexual. Growing up he had had only one boyfriend, a schoolmate he masturbated with up until the time the other guy got married, and only one "adult experience" in which he had been the one, he points out, who had fucked the other guy. The seminary turned into a turbulent experience, "just crisis after crisis," Jorge remembers. He told the priest assigned to be his confessor about the "adult experience," and also became very close to one of the other students, although there was no sex between them. Jorge was criticized for having made a "special friend," warned about it, then suddenly asked to leave the seminary. No reasons were given, and at first the fathers said his new friend would be allowed to come to the airport to see Jorge off. But at the last moment, permission was withdrawn.

I knew Jorge was also a friend of David Muna's, so I told him about David's warning me off Alejandro Guerrero. What was that all about? All I could imagine was that David must be terrified about SIDA, and somehow had Alejandro, the SIDA doctor, and maybe the Association as well, all mixed up with his fear and his own inability to *do* anything about it.

Maybe, Jorge said. His own explanation, however, was simpler. Poor David was given to sudden rages, to saying and doing things he didn't mean—driving customers out of his shop, yelling at them and frightening them. Not that David *meant* any of it, Jorge said. The best idea was not to pay much attention to some of the things he mouthed off about.

So as I was about to leave town yet one more time, I made a point of going back to say good-bye to David. This time, his visitor was a fellow named Ulises, beard, hairy chest, gray-green eyes, Hawaiian shirt. A grown daughter, David said. Ulises's birthday party was coming up on Saturday, and he was asking 150 people and bringing in three boy strippers from Cancún. I was invited.

I was sorry, I said, but my university wouldn't understand if I didn't show up to teach.

"Stay," David said. "Tell the *pinche* university that your grandmother left you a small inheritance, an *estancia* in Yucatán, and you had to go reconnoiter it."

Ulises's invitations were the kind sent out for children's birthday parties, teddy bears and rocking horses. Each one had an entrance card. The party wasn't going to be at his house, but at a friend's. "And you know how these queens are," he said. "If they hear about a free party, the discos will be empty that night." Each of the cards had a number on it, for the raffle.

"What's being raffled?" David asked.

"The strippers."

"Well, then give me ten numbers," David said, sticking out his hand, "I need them. I never win anything."

Baltazar is a waiter at the restaurant in one of the most elegant hotels, a client at Ya'ax Che, and Russell Rodriguez's patient at the T-1. I met him there one day in September 1992, when he had gotten off specially—usually he works seven to three, he told me, but today he'd gotten someone to change shifts with him—because he had run out of his medicine. "But now it turns out Dr. Russell isn't here," he said. "Maybe if I wait he will come back."

It is midday and no one else is in the clinic office, so we sit and talk quietly together in the cool and gloom. Baltazar has a shock of receding black hair with fine streaks of gray in it, which he brushes straight back, buffed nails, a soft, sweet style. He also has a dry throat, a little catlike cough he covers up by putting his pretty hand over his mouth. When from time to time he coughs up phlegm, he stops to spit it out into the potted plant by the door.

Baltazar was born in Mérida, though his mother and mother's family come from Motul. One of a large number of children, he still lives at home with his mother and two of his sisters. His other brothers and sisters don't even come to visit. His mother says, "Why don't they come to see me while I can still speak? What good will it be when they come and I'm dead?"

For a while, Baltazar had an apartment of his own, even though formally he was still living at home. This was because he was in a relationship with a married man. But the man eventually robbed him—tape-deck, television (which Baltazar calls a *tele* [tell-lay]—everything he owned.

He found out he was VIH-positive two years ago when his mother had to have surgery. She has hernias, diabetes, all sorts of problems. Baltazar gave blood at the hospital for his mother's operation. "What if they hadn't tested it?" he says. "What if they had put that blood in my mother?" He just shakes his head. It was lucky, that's all. He and his sister found a boy who *could* donate blood instead, and everything turned out all right.

Has he been sick? No, no problems at all so far, except for this little cough now, and some swelling in his tonsils. He's changed his life, Baltazar says, now he stays home in the evening, goes to church, reads passages from the Bible. He hasn't told anybody in his family. In fact not many people at all know, except of course the ones in his group. He's learned a lot from going to the self-help meetings at the Association, he says, from being with other people who have the disease.

"You look well," I say.

"Do I? How old do you think I am?"

Underestimating for his gray hair and papery skin, I say, "Fifty-two?"

Baltazar is forty-seven. To cover my embarrassment, I tell him well I'm fifty and he certainly looks a hundred times better than I do.

Oh no, he says, oh no—.

He tells about another affair he had with a married man, a young carpenter who noticed Baltazar smiling at him on a bus. The carpenter was twenty-four when they took up together. After a while, he had to go away to work in Cancún. Baltazar was able to go with him to the bus station to see him off. As a going-away present he brought the young man a pair of shorts he knew would look good on him. And afterward, when he'd come back to visit, the carpenter would not only go see his wife, he'd visit Baltazar as well. But then he was in a car accident and was killed.

I say, "There seem to be a lot of men around here who like other men, even those who are married."

"A lot," Baltazar agrees. "But many of them are very bad people, too. They keep asking you for things, they're only in it for what they can get off you. 'Buy me this watch, give me this shirt—' " He demonstrates plucking at my shirt, then laying his hand softly on my forearm. "When that man stole the *tele* from me—and it was a color *tele*, too—I went to his lawyer to complain. The lawyer said, 'But what are you going to do? He's already sold the television, and the tape machine, too,' and I said, 'Then he can give me the money he got.' Not that he ever did. He even had the nerve to come back to the apartment one time looking for me, but I told him, 'You're not welcome here, unless you've come prepared to give my things back first.' A dog, you give him something, you feed him, he'll come and kiss you and jump up into your arms. But this type of person, not even that—"

Then, as though he has warned me sufficiently about his countrymen, quite rapidly Baltazar moves to the subject of presents: "I just love giving people things, making them little gifts. If I see something I know my younger sister likes—a kind of perfume, say—I just buy it for her and give it to her, and there," flicking his nice hands at the imagined thing, "it gives me great pleasure to do that. Or to find something I think the doctors here might like, or José Manuel— They do so much for us, you know."

He hasn't told anyone at work about his condition. The other waiters are on you all the time, they don't any of them wish you well. The restaurant's maitre d' is a handsome young fellow who speaks English and French. He tells Baltazar he should pay him for sex, because he's really good. "But I tell him," Baltazar says, " 'I don't pay for it and I never have.' That guy has two little daughters he left behind in the D.F. I tell *him*, 'When you get a vacation, when you have the chance, you should go see your little girls.' 'But they're with their mother,' he tells me. And I tell him, 'If you have children, don't let them grow up without knowing their father. That's a sin.' "

Baltazar's own father died when he was twelve or thirteen.

Then in comes Elsa, the tall, sunny young woman who replaced Jenny as the office typist when Jenny went on maternity leave. Big hellos to both of us. Once she's at her own desk with her pocketbook beside her on the floor, she asks after Baltazar's mother. Oh, he says, Mother is the same, the same, a thousand aches and pains but with more life in her still than a lot of us certainly. "Last night do you know what she wanted to do, señorita? There was the parade downtown for the holiday and that lady wanted to go. Think of that." Baltazar laughs, then coughs a little. "Of course she couldn't go, not with her legs the way they are. But still—"

After a few minutes, Baltazar decides it's time for him to go try to find Dr. Russell again. Shaking hands, he lowers his voice again to remind me that I can always find him at the restaurant at the hotel, that he gets off at three.

The Captain's Touch

Alejandro tells me one day, "In Maya the word *coyaso* means a 'dip.' You are passing the bowl of chili and you scoop up a fingerful to eat, and that's a *coyaso*. Men will say about their friends, 'We are *coyasos*,' which means we take a dip from or we penetrate each other."

To the question of what's in a name, some of the anthropologists who trained me would certainly answer, "Everything." Proof of not only existence, but of the concept actually being functional in the minds of the people who use it. For the outsider a new term quickly becomes a puzzle piece that you hope may turn into a key that will let you into a larger reality about which you currently know nothing. I always liked watching the ethnographers experienced in field linguistics as they went about bringing forth some item from their current set of linguistic problems and laying it out for examination by one of those absolute authorities they call the "native speaker."

In my much less sophisticated methodology (here with a language I have almost no knowledge of), the first stop for my possible Mayan word for "sex buddies" was the Bookshop Dante in Hidalgo, where they have a copy of the gigantic, expensive 1980 Cordemex Dictionary of Yucatec Maya (as I recall it costs about a hundred dollars). There, alas, no *coyaso*, but at least a sound-alike root, a verb "*ko'oh*," which could mean "to dip."

(Later, back in the States, I called Victoria R. Bricker, an anthropologist and linguist now at Tulane whom I first knew almost thirty years ago when she was starting her graduate fieldwork in Chiapas. When we spoke, Victoria was in the process of finishing her own dictionary of Yucatec. She did not have any knowledge of the term I was worried about—but she was not against its possibility either, and told me the root *ko'oh* sounded to her like something borrowed by lowland Maya from Nahautl.)

My next stop was the busy old restaurant on the other side of the plaza called "The Louvre." Eating there from time to time, I had struck up a joking relationship with a dapper, broad-faced, tiny bustling sixty-ish gentleman who was one of the waiters. It had begun one day when I stood up next to him and one of the regulars asked him if I were his son. "Oh no," the waiter told everybody, standing closer to show off our enormous height disparity, "this is my *papi*!" Since then, it had become his habit always to welcome me as his "daddy," and mine to assure everyone that no, in our little family *he* was the daddy. As my friend ran among the tables, he would also test my knowledge of—mostly sexual—words and phrases in Maya (the word for penis, the one for vagina, how to ask a woman how much it would cost to sleep with her). The evening I asked him what *ko'ohaso* (as I was now spelling it) might mean, he was especially busy. He started away from my table and I thought maybe he hadn't heard me. But then he wheeled around and said, "*Ko'ohaso*? You know," and stuck out his middle finger and made jabbing motions as though he was goosing somebody, raised his eyebrows, laughed, and hurried on.

So at least Mayan men joke about having anal intercourse with each other. Beyond this "fact," however, I was left with only questions. How frequently does anal sex between men actually occur? Under what circumstances? What other sexual acts do Mayan men talk about doing with one another? Is there affection involved? Pressure? Shame? Are their sexual relationships likely to be short- or long-term? How much do Mayan women know about what their men do together? What are their own lives with other women like? What sort of connections do homosexuality and heterosexuality have for Mayan people?

It was only a while after my talk with Baltazar at the T-1 that I realized I might have asked him what he knew about *ko'ohasos*. In Mérida, at least for gringos and other foreigners, it is not at all obvious who might be Mayan or who still speaks the language. The movement into the city from the surrounding country in the last decades has been epic in scope, but, as a migration, it has not been complete. The road to Mérida (like the one to Cancún) still runs both ways. Though Baltazar was born in the city, when he tells me his family is from Motul, he *may* mean that he still has ties to the historic town, goes there to visit relatives, observes religious holidays there, speaks some Maya himself. Many men and boys work six days every week where the jobs are, in Mérida or in Cancún, then go home to their families from Saturday afternoon to Monday morning. Though there are an estimated 400,000 Mayan speakers in the state, some sociologists at the university say that the language is in decline. Certainly, more and more Mayan people need to be fluent in Spanish in order to make a living, and radio and television and the teaching of Spanish in even the smallest villages enable more children to grow up with two languages that they can use as needed. Often, adults will tell you that they have completely forgotten their Maya, though what they mean is that they feel "rusty" in it. As soon as they go among Mayan speakers again, it comes back.

Whites (Spanish speakers) tend to claim that the division between the two cultures has lost significance and that the Yucatán is a single society now, the distinction between themselves and the Maya a matter of race and heritage, yes, but not of *race-ism* or prejudice. Basically, an urban-rural division, they would say, the Maya a historically willing peasantry responsive to white leadership in matters regarding money, planning, and any dealings with the greater world beyond the peninsula. Two coexistent cultures, the whites maintain, full of mutual respect and fondness for each other. After all, in their closets the governor and all the wealthiest ladies of Mérida keep richly embroidered silk versions of the mestiza's humble cotton *huipil*, which they trot out for all the social occasions where the *Jarana* is danced and the sovereignty of Yucatán is celebrated.

The division between Mayan and white *is* urban-rural, but there is also a class distinction and a language/ethnicity division marked by antagonism on both sides and, historically, by a will to separation at any cost on the part of at least some of the Maya. The whites' version of a happy integration out of necessity glides over the bloody Caste War of the nineteenth century and ignores the fact that well into the twentieth Mayan rebels from the hacienda system continued proclaiming themselves a separate nation in Quintana Roo. The confusion that outsiders like me experience in telling who is Mayan and who is white never seems a problem for those born in the peninsula. Every interaction between members of the two groups—every slight, every condescension, every aside in the language that the other may not understand—reaffirms their differences. At some level, each side also subscribes to the theory that the other is unknowable. This common belief allows both white and Mayan to remain ignorant of each other in important ways, despite their having lived side by side for five hundred years.

While the city still drew most of its wealth from the countryside, the whites continued to take at least a proprietary interest in the well-being of the Maya. As long as henequén remained a slow but excellent cash producer, they managed their haciendas and spent some of their time living on them. But now, since the sudden death of the sisal market, they have abandoned the country to the Maya, saying, in effect, "Here, you always claimed this territory was yours. Now that it is worthless, you can have it back." The low productivity of the land these days is also used as justification for the neglect of those who try to live off it. In the whites' version of things, Indian people's constant malnutrition and their occasional flirtation with starvation are their own fault. They have been intransigent, bent on keeping their old ways, and so have fallen irreparably far behind while the other segments of society have waged the heroic struggle to bring Mexico into the First World. As a result of the new fabulation, the PRI may install a sleek new cement basketball court in the plaza in the weeks before an election, but despite the television advertisements for the glories of the party's *Solidaridad* program, new electricity, potable water, and sewage programs are seldom offered anymore to the smaller towns. In most questions concerning health, whites feel justified in their abandonment of the country.

In 1976 I spent the winter months living outside a village called Chelem on the coast north of Mérida and west of the deep-dredged ports at Progreso and Yukalpetén. The Gulf of Mexico here is a smoky lime green, the flow of the tide east-west. At night sometimes the sea becomes so placid you can see the moon in it whole. Phosphorus glows in the small churn along the waterline. There are coconut palms with green-yellow nuts and nests of birds and scorpions in their upper reaches, iguanas burrowing in the warm sand.

Hipolito Pech Mena, a Chelem fisherman who worked for me part of the time that winter, was convinced that coastal Mayan people have a singular advantage over their inland kin. "Living here by the sea," Polito would say, "we will never starve." (This was in the time before the big petroleum spills in the Gulf, the natural gas leak fires burning on top of the water, and the coming of the big international fishing ships to take away the baby shrimp.) Boats owned or part-owned by men in the villages still went out, taking a crew of nine or ten and carrying enough ice to pack their catch in for between a week and ten days. Though most specialized in shrimp, they brought in a variety of fish as well, *mero*, *robalo*, *huachinango*, *cazón* (grouper, bass, red snapper, dogfish). No one but the captains and the landbound co-owners of the boats made enough money to save anything, but at least the enterprise was satisfying, long shifts of skilled work with a few hours sleep on deck in-between, and full of adventure. Many men in Chelem knew the ports of Galveston, New Orleans, and Tampico, and most of them had been stranded or sunk or knocked overboard at one time or another, or blown onto the southern shores of Cuba, 131 miles to the northeast of the Yucatán. Sudden loss, the unpredictability of the elements, and salvation from unexpected sources were all themes of their stories.

Anthropologists generally press the nuclear family as the cornerstone of social organization in Mayan Yucatán. They recognize that work is almost completely divided up along gender lines, but fail to emphasize that the division means, in practice, that men spend most of their time among men, and women with women. In Chelem, fishing, boat and net repair, land clearing, and corn raising were male tasks; women washed, cooked, and cared for babies and children and the home. Your familial relationships were very important in both work and leisure life (who you "are," what jobs you may get, even where your house is located are all defined by who you were kin with), but even on social occasions the sexes still kept fairly much apart from each other.

The result made it seem sometimes as though there were really two distinct communities. I would sense it strongly when Polito and I went into Progreso, the port town forty-five minutes by bus from Chelem. There was a large popular restaurant downtown on the corner of the plaza where we would eat. The more time I spent there, the more obvious it became how separate men's business was from women's. Living side by side, congenial, mutually respectful, with interests in one another's affairs—their children, for example, and sexual matters—but otherwise quite exclusive. Though women were certainly welcome, the restaurant was principally a men's place. Groups began forming early in the morning for coffee, people came and went, old gentlemen poked their heads in at the big open doors to see if there was anyone inside they wanted to sit and chat with. It went on all day, and up until nine or ten in the evening when the restaurant closed. Among women, the younger ones came in to eat in pairs, the older ones in bigger groups with children and grandchildren in tow. When middle-class families from Mérida or beyond entered and took tables, their more gender-integrated style, the focus on attending to the men, no matter what their age, put the two-society distinction I thought I saw among the local people in even sharper contrast.

At the time I had not read Landa's *Relación de las cosas de Yucatan* (1566), so I did not know about the bishop's claim about the existence of separate men's houses in the time before the Conquest. (The *Relación* is a schizophrenic piece of work. Written in Spain while Landa was under indictment for the excessive brutality of his administration in the New World, it is above all an apologia where the lurid and abominable paganism of the Maya serves as justification for the author's actions. But it is also obvious that Landa cherishes the memory of the culture he tried to crush and that at one point he must have worked very hard to learn everything he could about it. As a result, the *Relación* functions in two registers, elegy and denunciation, often going back and forth from one to the other sentence by sentence.) Landa's claim is that, before the arrival of the Spanish, out of "respect" for their elders the young men did not mingle with them, except on occasions of necessity, like weddings. "Also," he says,

> they visited little among married people; so that it was the custom to have in each town a large building, whitewashed and open on all sides, where the young men gathered for their pastimes. They played ball, and a certain game with beans like dice, and many others. Here they nearly always slept, all together, until they were married.[8]

Landa goes on immediately to assure his reader that the young men were never "guilty of unnatural offenses in these houses" (he means sodomy), which he notes has been reported for other societies of the Indies. His proof is that "they say that those addicted to this pestilential vice care nothing for women, as these people did." In fact, according to Landa, the men brought female prostitutes into their separate dwellings and the women, though compensated, were "so beset by the number of the youths that they were harassed even to death."

I do not know what to make of the claim about the prostitutes dying from overwork. It seems impossible, and perhaps only reflective of Landa's bizarre zealotry in his believing it enough to report it. What interests me is the description of a marked homosocial life for men before marriage, and Landa's sixteenth-century understanding that what is homosocial is not *necessarily* homosexual.

In Chelem, at the end of the day I would walk the kilometer or so into town and go drink beer with the fishermen I knew out under the thatched roof of an open-air bar a half block from the beach. For a while I was a novelty. "California, think of that," they would say. One of the people who would come by, usually later on, was captain of one of the Chelem boats, a curly-haired man in his late thirties. He took a special interest in me. He would always pull a chair over next to mine, and when it was dark and we had all had a good deal of beer, he would put his hand under the table and rub my knee. Once or twice I let my hand go over onto his knee.

Hard to believe now, but at the time I had no idea what to do next. The captain was married (I met his wife and children one time, at a christening while he was out fishing). Would we have walked back all the way to the place I was staying? Or gone down by the water, under the palm trees? Drunk, we had trouble understanding each other. Maybe I completely misinterpreted the whole thing.

Chuburná Puerto, the village beyond Chelem to the west, has a small medical clinic. One of the young *pasantes* assigned there in 1988 and 1989 was a woman named Karla Beatriz Uribe Martínez. For her MD thesis, Karla Uribe conducted a survey in Spanish of fifty women and fifty men of reproductive age (fourteen to forty-five), which is the only piece of research so far concerning SIDA among Mayan people of Mexico. The result, "Knowledge of a Fishing Community Concerning the Problem of SIDA," bears dedications to Uribe's advisers, Dr. Renán Góngora-Biachi and Dr. Pedro González-Martínez. Her principal "finding" is that men and women in Chuburná Puerto have only what she calls a "regular" understanding of SIDA, gained mostly from radio and television. They know that SIDA is a sexually transmitted disease. Sixty-one percent cite "promiscuous sex" as the means of contagion. Asked to name one method of prevention, 40 percent of both men and women said avoiding extramarital heterosexual relations. Another 40 percent of the men mentioned avoiding homosexual relationships, while 30 percent of women said "avoiding physical contact." (Eight percent of women named "using prophylactics" as a prevention, but no men cited that method.)

Uribe's second major "finding" is that the people she interviewed think homosexuality is frequent in Yucatán (she means male homosexuality). Eighty-eight percent of men and 62 percent of women claimed to know at least one homosexual. When given the choices of "acceptance," "indifference," or "rejection" as possible attitudes toward homosexuality, 74 percent of women chose rejection, 18 percent chose indifference. Among men, though, 52 percent chose indifference, and 44 percent rejection. (Only four women and two men favored acceptance.) When asked to estimate what percentage of young men between fourteen and twenty they thought had had sex with another boy or man at least once, nearly half of both women and men imagined the range to be somewhere between 20 and 40 percent. A majority of men (64 percent) said they had been invited to "attend homosexual gatherings," but only 2 percent (i.e., one man) admitted to having accepted such an invitation.

Karla Uribe offers no account of the discrepancies between the men's estimates of the homosexual activities of *other* men and what they say about their own experience. From her data, it would appear that many are propositioned but few are actually seduced. (Uribe also asked for estimates of the percentage of young women between fourteen and twenty who have had "at least one sexual experience [not of a homosexual type]," but she does not include answers to this question in her thesis. Her focus was clearly not on sexual life in its variety, but on establishing possible routes of transmission of SIDA.) Uribe's questions about numbers of "homosexual experiences" *may* be framed well enough to get reasonable answers, but her idea of what "male homosexuality" means may not be what the citizens of Chuburná Puerto understand it to mean when they try to respond to her. For them, the Spanish noun *homosexual* probably conjures up a man, perhaps a bachelor (but perhaps married too), maybe an occasional cross-dresser, who is known in the community to be available for sex with other men. But the term *male homosexuality* may not include for them the experience of a husband and father who had anal intercourse with other boys before he married or who continues to have sex with other men when he is out on a fishing boat. Why do more men say they are "indifferent" to it and more women that they "reject" it? How much is the women's "rejection" a response based on what they know the Church and white people like Dr. Uribe expect good Catholics and upright citizens like themselves to say?

Are the people of Chuburná Puerto right? Is homosexual experience fairly common among Mayan men? (Or is sex between men perhaps more common in *coastal* regions? There is a good-sized inland town directly east of Mérida called Tixkokob where, it is said, at one point the entire *ayuntamiento*, or local government, was made up of homosexuals. From its gay reputation, Tixkokob is sometimes called *el Puerto Seco* [the Dry Port].)

Native people of the Yucatán are said to be as thoroughly "studied" as any in the world except certain southwestern U.S. Indian groups. But the anthropological record on subjects of sexuality in general is slim, and what there is about homosexuality is contradictory. In a book published in 1931, the ethnologist T.W.F. Gann says of the people in neighboring British Honduras, "Both men and women are singularly lacking in sex instinct, and this seems to have been a characteristic of the Maya from the earliest times."[9] Robert Redfield, whose 1941 *The Folk Culture of Yucatán*, and later *A Village That Chose Progress: Chan Kom Revisited*, set the standard for small-community ethnographies for several decades, mentions that a woman in one village is thought to be a lesbian, but has nothing further to offer about homosexuality for either sex. In the 1960s anthropologist Irwin Press studied Pustunich, a community of about a thousand at the time he was there. "Homosexuality is known," Press says (he means among men), "and all agree that there is none in Pustunich . . ." However, Press also tells us that there are said to be "four or five" homosexuals in nearby Ticul, a town of fifteen thousand, and that in Pustunich itself "a soft-featured catrín boy of ten is suspected of future potential." (In rural Yucatán, a *catrín* is a person who emphasizes white over Mayan culture, speaking Spanish and wearing "city" or Western-style clothes.) On the other hand, one man interviewed by anthropologist Walter Williams for his book *The Spirit and the Flesh* maintains unequivocally, "There are some homosexuals in every Maya village."[11]

Williams's account is based on a month's visit to the Yucatán in 1983. He did not know Maya, but had the advantage of having as his traveling companion a young man who did. Williams himself is committed to the theories of what are sometimes called the essentialists, who believe that homosexual men universally constitute a "third sex" with special religious or spiritual status wherever they appear in traditional culture. Williams follows the practice of differentiating between "men" or "males" (meaning heterosexual men) and "homosexuals." In Yucatán, he says, *homosexuales* take "the passive role in either anal or oral sex, and are considered the true homosexual." Their "masculine" boyfriends have "no sense of identity as homosexuals," so they bear "no burden of being labeled 'abnormal,' because in fact their behavior is normal for that society." Most men keep to the role they assign themselves. Yet, Williams adds,

> Passive homosexuals have told me of instances where their *hombre* boyfriends played the passive role in sex, but this was done only after a level of trust had been established so that such role reversals would be kept secret. Sex with a male is not something to be embarrassed about, but role reversal is.[12]

In one small town a man in his mid-twenties whose nickname was "El Sexy" told Williams that men would ask him to dance at the local cantina and that during the festivities at Carnaval, when he dressed as a woman, he was "especially popular" as a dance partner:

> The other people appreciate me very much. Because I behave properly. *Hombres* will have sex with each other when they get drunk, but I consider that to be bad. It should only be done with an *homosexual*, then it's all right. I would not have sex with another *homosexual*; I don't consider them to be completely men. They're like a third group, different from men or women.[13]

He told Williams that he had "had relations with most of the men in his village, from teenagers to the elderly. 'They know I'm good,' he remarks." El Sexy lived with his mother, so he wouldn't bring men home for sex. They would usually go behind the church or out in the village's sports field.

Another *homosexual* Williams met was a prosperous forty-year-old man who dressed "in a mixture of men's and women's clothing" and owned a popular beauty shop in a town in the southern part of the state. The day Williams talked with him, the man had his hair up in pink rollers and was giving a "middle-aged proper-looking woman" a manicure:

> Everyone knows I'm *homosexual*, and I am well respected. There are hundreds of *homosexuales* in town, most openly so, but I am the only one who dresses as a woman. The people treat me as a woman, and there are never any problems. I attend mass devotedly; the priest often visits my house for meals because I'm one of the best cooks in town. People respect my good citizenship. The men come to visit me for sex; I have to turn them away. I had a lover for several years, and we walked around town holding hands being com-

pletely open. No one objects. I feel no discrimination for being different.[14]

In highland Chiapas, Mayan men dress up as women for certain religious fiestas where they join a company of other larger-than-life figures—monkeys, conquistadores, batmen, jaguars, spooks, clowns—to act out well-known, long-handed-down dramatic scenarios. In drag, Indian men get the chance to burlesque higher station *ladinos* (whites) by imitating their women.[15] They make fun of the elevated members of their own community, too, chiding male officials for improper performance of duty and men and women for inordinate sexual "heat." Unusual and inappropriate appetite in sex—heterosexual or homosexual—is a theme of transvestites' parody in the Yucatán as well as in Chiapas. In the highlands, taking a female role in religious fiestas carries no connotation about a man's sexuality in daily life. The village *travesti* of Yucatán, cross dressing year-round and widely known as an available homosexual, does not seem to exist as a regular figure in the highlands.

In 1965 I visited in Ticul where the anthropologist Duane Metzger had a field station. Another gringo was also working there, not connected with Duane, a quiet, balding bachelor psychologist from some other university. For a big dance—maybe it was Valentine's Day—the men in the neighborhood, shoemakers, fixed the psychologist up with a date. "She" was so well done, the shoemakers told Duane, that the psychologist passed the entire evening at the *Club de Leones* without ever finding out he was dancing and flirting with another man.

Ten years later I caught sight of drags (whether Mayan or white I couldn't tell) in Progreso during *Carnaval*. A dinky, noisy little daytime parade was marching down the main thoroughfare and there they were, across the street and ahead, three or four big, loud made-up beauty queens in wigs, diving into the crowd and kissing people, but then running (at least one in heels) to keep up with the line of march and the slouching older convertibles they were supposed to be riding in.

Hocabá is a town 27 kilometers southeast of Mérida. There, at Carnaval, the *travestis* enact a drama in Maya which Victoria Bricker has described.[16] The play is about a man named Juan Carnaval, "the villain of the fiesta," and "Mariquita, the star female impersonator" of the occasion, who "pretends to be a homosexual." After escaping from jail, Juan Carnaval is apprehended and brought up before a judge. His accomplices, it appears, have all been "artists" (homosexuals or transvestites) from the Zona de Tolerancia (the old redlight district of Mérida, closed down twenty years ago). The place Juan Carnaval has run off to is Progreso. There is talk about him going down in the ocean and an encounter with a *b'usóob'*, which means both a "diver" and a homosexual, and with "crabs" (*haib'aób*), also a term for homosexuals. Asked if he isn't ashamed to be seen with such people, Juan Carnaval tells the judge, "No, sir, because if it were not for them, I would be dead now from hunger, because my wives don't work to support me. The little crabs, on the other hand, even buy me chewing gum."

The message of the incident seems quite clear. If women do not do exactly what is expected of them, their husbands may resort to urban homosexuals—who *do* desire them—not only for their pleasures, but for their sustenance as well.

Because of a particular Mayan double standard, the linguists and ethnographers who have learned the language have found out far more about the texture of sexual life than other outsiders have been able to glean. Children, girls especially, are brought up to be extremely modest, and adult men and women remain very concerned about one another's sexual arrangements. Yet, adult conversation is filled with constant sexual joking. Men seem to engage in it more than women, but women indulge as well. Flowing all in Maya, seldom overheard by outsiders, sexual talk is one element of what continues as the secret life of the society.[17]

One of the subjects men joke with each other about is sex among themselves. Anthropological linguist William F. Hanks offers several examples. Here is one:

> AB, an adult man, is walking towards the market early in the morning when he sees TG, a familiar, passing on a bicycle. The exchange takes places as TG passes, without slowing:
>
> AB: Hey TG, will you take me along? (= can you take my whole penis?)
>
> TG: Sure, get up (on the back of the bike). (= sure, just try and jump on me).
>
> AB: You'll shit on me.[18]

The same two men may also get a laugh from a group by boasting that they are having sex with each other's wives. Hanks points out, however, that these exchanges require utter discretion. Outside of joking situations, friends like AB and TG are likely to be too discreet even to admit that they ever even *met* each other's spouses.

Georgina Martínez, the director of the Asociación Ya'ax Che, sent a brief proposal for educating Mayan women about SIDA to the governor of the state. The plan would put some funds into the development of educational materials—posters, maybe handouts—for distribution in places like Hocabá, Chuburná Puerto, Pustunich, and Chelem. But the proposal's main idea was to organize groups that would train key local women, such as *comadronas* (midwives), who could then pass along information about the virus and safer sex to other women. The cost of the program for a year would be U.S. $30,000, and would include developing and printing the educational materials, transportation to the villages, and full or partial salary for the three people to be employed in the project.

The governor rejected Georgina's proposal. As a sociologist the governor's judgment was that it wouldn't work. Mayan women's famous modesty about sexual matters, she said, would keep them from ever talking about such matters in groups.

The obstacle the governor points out definitely exists. Barbara Holmes, a student of Victoria Bricker at Tulane, learned Maya and wrote a dissertation based primarily on her work with women in Hocabá in the early seventies. Both men and women, she writes, "distrust each other and their own sexuality. Their bodies are shameful. They assiduously avoid all instruction about physiology. Their shame is a source of vulnerability, especially at moments of elimination and procreation. These are the body functions that leave them physically exposed; these are the situations that are laughed at."[19]

In the village of Chan Kom, ethnographer Mary Elmendorf confirmed the commonplace that Mayan women do not even pass on information about menstruation to their daughters. She then asked her friend "Anita" whether she had spoken to her nearly grown daughter about what to expect concerning sex once she became an adult:

ANITA: No.
ELMENDORF: Shouldn't you?
ANITA: No—it's a sin.
ELMENDORF: Won't she be surprised by a man sometime? . . . and she won't know what's happening. Or when she marries?
ANITA: (Laughs.) Well, when you marry it is very surprising because you don't know.[20]

Elmendorf found, however, that as an outsider she was free to talk with women about how they could get birth control materials, and that the women were glad to have the information she could give them.

The real problem with Georgina's proposal is also its great advantage: it would establish situations where discussion—learning—about the risks of SIDA might actually take place, but it does not promise the kind of tangible "product" that the people with money to spend want to see. Village midwives may not have advanced degrees in public health, but they remain the preferred authorities and helpers to whom women turn when they are going to give birth.[21] As a group, *comadronas* seem quite independent, capable of balancing traditional beliefs with their own changing sense of what is best for their clients. In recent years, for example, they have become advocates of family planning, despite what they know to be the Catholic Church's position on the subject.

For an equivalent educational program for men and boys, it would be necessary to find out who among men has the authority that a midwife has with women. (The anthropological references to traditional education of women about sex are few; about men, I have found none.) It might turn out to be easy to get men to use condoms when they have sex with each other. The "indifference" toward homosexuality that the fishermen of Chuburná Puerto expressed to young Dr. Uribe may have been a subtle way of referring to its virtues. They know that the Church and the whites, and maybe their wives, are against it, but sex between men has been a pleasure that both parties involved *choose* (there are no reports of male rape in the towns and villages). In the days before SIDA, between men there were none of the possible unpleasant consequences that could lie in relations with women—no babies, no irate parents demanding they get married, no cuckholded husband seeking retribution. And, in the sexual realm, what is most "casual" may be the thing most amenable to change.

It might turn out to be easy—

My friend Matú tells me he is working on his own book about SIDA. For the front cover, he plans to have himself photographed in a *manta* shirt with no collar, drawstring pants, and *huaraches*, the costume of a man from the countryside. "No one in the *extranjero* will get it," he says. "They think we're all Indians down here anyway." Matú will begin by explaining he is a *campesino* who has been having sex with his best friend for a number of years. But now he's heard a little about this SIDA business and he thinks maybe his friend even has it, so he's come to the city to learn how to protect himself. The point, of course, will be to show how little the poor man will be able to find out in Mérida.

Independently, without knowing Matú's idea, I had been working on a similar fantasy. Everyone tells me prophylactics are readily available here. So around noon on a Saturday, still the big market day in Mérida, I visit the two large pharmacies on the south side of the main plaza. Both stores are crowded. The first features cosmetics, perfumes, and soaps for women and men in display cases at the front of the store, with the pharmacy in the back. The other is smaller and has Band-Aids and toothpaste and aspirin on open racks for the customer to select and bring to the cashier. In neither place do I see any condoms on display. I assume you could ask for them from the clerks who handle the prescriptions.

What do they cost in stores? In another part of the country I saw a packet of three for 7,000 pesos—U.S. $2.25.

One evening I go looking for a water-based lubricant jelly. I try two of the *supermercados* downtown near the main market. These are large, busy, open-front emporiums with butchers' counters in the back, a version of fast food (pots of carry-out *mole*), and large sections devoted to soap, shampoos, conditioners, gel, men's hair oil, other lotions for the hair, men's and women's deodorants, racks of aerosol shaving soap, razor blades, baby oil, high towers of paper diapers. No home pregnancy testing kits, no sexual lubricants at all, not even Vaseline, no spermicides, and no condoms.

Several blocks away in a "real" pharmacy with a counter and the goods stacked on shelves behind it, I ask the young woman if they have a *tubo de lubricante sexual.* She doesn't seem to understand me. One brand name in the States, I tell her, is "K-Y." She goes to get a somewhat older male employee, maybe the pharmacist. He disappears and in a while comes back with a big tube of something called "Lubrizal," a *jalea lubricante* that contains 0.1 percent *Cloro de Benalconio* as its active ingredient, the rest "*vehiculo.*" Whether the Lubrizal is water-based I can't tell from the tube (experimenting with it later I found that it was). I assume it doesn't contain nonoxydol 9. It cost 5,800 pesos, slightly under U.S. $2.00.

As my search becomes a regular game, the wholesale emporiums around the market begin to look a bit sinister to me. All that stuff sold on counters in little stores in little towns all over the peninsula, cheap hard candy, plastic toys, the nipples for bottles, all the varieties of formula, all the perfumy, pricy scents meant to make people irresistible to one another. But none of the things they need to protect themselves sexually. *Preservativos. Condones. Jalea lubricante.* Even if that man in from the country had the money to spare and knew what to ask for *and* believed the strange, almost unbelievable story about how the wretched sickness is passed and how long it can remain hidden in your blood, he would still have to deal with the impatient young ladies behind the counter and wait to get a private word with the pharmacist to ask him to make a special trip to get the things out of wherever it is he has them stashed away.

THE VISITORS FROM WAKAX

SEPTEMBER 1992

I will call the town Wakax (pronounced Wa-KASH). It lies to the northeast, an hour and forty-five minutes outside Mérida on the bus, beyond Motul in what is called the "henequén zone." Originally, Wakax was one of the great haciendas with its own mill for processing cactus spears into fiber. Almost thirty years ago the operation—what was left of it—was turned over to the people who live there. Today, Wakax is both a town of six thousand and a collectively held *ejido*.

Six cases so far, Alejandro tells me when I return to Mérida at the end of the first week in September. One was a homosexual, he came from somewhere else, kept a kitchen, a kind of restaurant, had relations with other homosexuals and bisexual men. Last week he died, here in the T-1. Wakax is large enough to have a secondary school. Two teachers there are seropositive. They have told José Manuel and Alejandro that they have been having sex with some of their male students. Among the cases so far is one young woman whose husband is also positive. They have two children, six and ten, both of whom have been brought in for the VIH test. The children have shown up negative.

All these discoveries in the last four months.

Wakax is fairly near the Gulf coast. In the next town beyond it are female prostitutes, many of whose customers are fishermen who come in to see them when they are paid off after a trip out to sea. Several years ago Renán Góngora-Biachi and his colleagues took blood samples from the registered prostitutes in this second town and only one woman tested seropositive. Now Alejandro wonders if there will be a route of SIDA transmission from the men of Wakax to the prostitutes of the second town and out into the world via the fishermen.

One per thousand is not a high incidence of infection if you compare Wakax, for example, to the gay male community in San Francisco, where one in two is HIV-positive. But for a small town, where there is no anonymity, where gossip rules—Alejandro also wonders how his office is going to let people's families know what is happening and get them to come to Mérida to be tested without spreading panic or compromising the two schoolteachers.

There is one especially cruel wrinkle in this already cruel situation. In the last several years IMSS has been purging its rolls. Six months ago workers in henequén lost their full *vigente* status with IMSS. There were abuses, Alejandro says, people using one another's cards, using cards belonging to people who had died or gone off to work in the States. Now henequén worker families are entitled only to the "basic" or "level-one" services the system offers (in Wakax, this means the attention they can get at the small IMSS clinic there). The husband and wife who are seropositive are thus no longer entitled to the stipend that would enable them to get to Mexico City for a T helper cell test, or to the test itself. The catch is that without proof of a T helper ratio of less than five hundred, they cannot receive AZT through IMSS. (Whether Alejandro and Russell would be allowed to put them on an antiviral if they somehow managed to get tested on their own I do not know.)

As we are talking about it, Alejandro gets a phone call. When he hangs up, he announces that the administration is willing to allow the couple to receive the T cell test for free. They have never been to Mexico City themselves, but they have a relative who has and who could accompany them. The remaining stumbling block is the funds to get all three to the D.F., and to feed and lodge them there overnight.

Russell arrives in his long white coat. "Charlie! I wasn't expecting you!" He shakes my hand, gives me a little *abrazo*. "How long are you here for?"

"Only two weeks."

"You come and go too often, Charlie. You ought to come and stay six months."

"I'd like to. But my work won't let me off and—" I can't remember whether I have told Russell about Ray being HIV-positive.

"And?"

"My lover doesn't trust me."

Russell starts nodding sympathetically. "He knows you then," he says.

Alejandro's other news is that he is in some trouble as a result of a talk he gave in August to a group of doctors about safer sex. At the end of the session, audience members asked for copies of the "information" so they could have it handy to use in advising their homosexual patients. (Why that in particular? Could they not admit that the heterosexual part of the information wasn't at their fingertips? Or was it that the same-sex part was so truly new and impressive to them?) They would keep it right there on their desks as reference, they promised Alejandro.

What he had presented came from a thousand-word pamphlet distributed by CONASIDA, which Alejandro showed me. From the content, the target audience seems to be fairly general—sexually active people, straight, gay, and bisexual. The advice offered is straightforward: whatever the sex of your partner, use condoms during intercourse, either vaginal or anal; use a water-based lubricant. Otherwise, it is not a very technical document (no sex organs pictured, not a how-to-put-on-a-condom piece). Exploration and mutual satisfaction are stressed—another person's body as a territory to be learned, giving pleasure as a pleasure in itself.

Instead of sending off for more copies of the pamphlet, Alejandro had most of the text copied and sent out to the doctors in mimeograph form, without any attribution to CONASIDA. For his trouble, he received a letter from the director of Public Health for the state of Yucatán. Alejandro was told he was "out of control" and "lacking discipline," that documents such as the one he had promulgated would actually *promote* homosexuality and, bottom line, that he was not to make any further public statements or issue anything else in writing that had not received prior explicit approval from *Salud Publica*.

What is really disturbing them about the material? First, I think, the fact that the sexuality of the *audience* for the pamphlet is not specified. "Bear these things in mind *whoever* you're having sex with" is the implication. No moral line is drawn between gay and straight. The other truly disquieting message may be the one about give and take, the ideal of learning how to gratify your partner, whether the partner is a man or a woman. "Mutuality" has become a commonplace of sex manuals and the stuff of thousands of magazine articles not only in the United States but in Mexico as well. Yet it is not hard to imagine how unsettling the theme could be to middle-aged male medical professionals, especially those who see it as part of their job to defend the existing social order.

Alejandro knows the doctor who passed the offending mimeograph along to the public health director. He is a colleague at the T-1 and head of one of the services where Alejandro reports. The man's brother is VIH-positive and Alejandro's patient.

Alejandro went to see the other doctor. "You chose to go behind my back," he told him, "but I'm coming to *you* directly, face to face." On the wall the other doctor had framed photographs of the Pope and Mother Teresa. "In the end," Alejandro said, "you know, *I'm* going to be the one to have my picture up there with them, because *I'm* the one who's acting like the Christian missionary in this situation, while you—"

His colleague told him he couldn't believe Alejandro would make such a comparison.

"You must have been pretty angry," I tell Alejandro.

He smiles, shrugs. "I suppose I was."

What will happen? He doesn't know yet. Maybe the conservatives, the Catholics, the Pro-Life doctors, will continue complaining and have him relieved of the directorship of the Office of Anti-SIDA Activities. If they do, Alejandro says, he can always simply devote himself to his clinical practice with VIH-positive patients, a turn of circumstances he would actually enjoy.

And he does have allies with some power. His friends more closely involved with politics have promised to see what can be done.

At *comida* at the restaurant across the street, I meet Alejandro's beautiful seventeen-year-old daughter Aleida for the first time. She has come back from Cancún to live with her father in the little house behind the actor's because the high schools in Mérida have the courses she needs to finish up and get into the university. Her classes begin in the afternoon, so she studies at home in the morning, then comes to eat with her father on her way to her "*prepa.*"

Coming back across the T-1 plaza, the concrete dazzling in the sun, Alejandro nods to fellow doctors going past and stops to say hello and shake hands with young women secretaries, assistants, nurses. To me, in a lowered voice: "What they *say* is the problem with me is that I don't fit in—I'm 'inappropriate' for this work because I've been married so many times. Or because I'm not married at the moment. Or because my life isn't what they call 'orderly.' "

Twenty-four hours later, paying our check at the restaurant, saying good-bye to Aleida, hurrying a bit to get back to the office, out on the sidewalk we met up with Miguel, one of the patients hospitalized in March when I was here. With him is his mother. Big hellos and handshakes all around.

"You're looking very well," I say.

"Thank you," says Miguel. "I am well."

His mother nodding, big smile, eyes darting back and forth between us and her boy. We say good-bye.

Miguel is nearly six feet, much taller than I imagined (I had not seen him standing up before). In the five months since his pneumonia episode he has put on a good deal of weight. I did not lie about how he looked. But his skin is much darker now, that uniform nut color people with HIV sometimes become, like a bad makeup job for an amateur Othello.

Alejandro, Russell, and José Manuel do not often volunteer information about patients I have met before. Part professional discretion, I assume, part their being busy with current problems, part the need not to look back. This afternoon, alone in the office with José Manuel, I suddenly decide the best possible moment has arrived, so I move over and sit across from him at his desk. "May I ask something?"

"Anything, Carter." José Manuel bats his eyes at me. "You know that."

"There were two patients—I would like to know what happened to them after I left."

"Yes, Carter, of course. Who?"

"Our friend Juanito, and the patient Jorge Dario Valle."

The second name does not seem to register immediately with José Manuel, so I add, "The man with syphilis. His sister is a nurse here."

"Oh yes." José Manuel nods, turns in his chair and brings down his ledger book, opens it, begins flipping the worn pages. "When did you go?"

"The thirtieth of March."

"They died, Carter. Juanito—" he looks, "—the thirty-first, and Jorge Dario—the thirtieth it appears. Maybe while you were in the air."

José Manuel continues letting the long pages drop, looking here and there while he reminisces a little about Juanito. What good friends they were, from well before the time Juanito ever got sick. What fine skin he had and how he cared for it.

"Did he go about as a *travesti*?" I ask. "In the streets?"

"Not always, no."

"Were you lovers at some point?"

"Well, not really. A little. Juanito always wanted someone who could buy him things, take care of him," José Manuel laughs, "and that wasn't ever going to be me, so—"

All week Alejandro and Russell sail in and out of the SIDA clinic in their white coats, neither of them inviting me to come up and see what's happening on the wards. There has been an outbreak of cholera in the town of Umán, which is on the road to both Uxmal and Campeche. So far, 150 cases have been reported. IMSS has a thirty-bed clinic in Umán, but they have run out of space and medicine, and are sending the overflow to Mérida. The sick arrive at all hours of the day and night in taxis or in private cars.

Processions from the villages were coming to pay their respects to the powerful Virgin of Umán, parades provided by *gremios*, voluntary organizations based on the old model of craft guilds and devoted to making the fiestas of particular saints (elsewhere they are sometimes called *cofradías*). As part of the celebration they made up and distributed large quantities of *horchata*, the sweet white rice powder drink, using water from *pozos* (wells) that turned out to be tainted. The reports are extravagant, the scene described medieval, with modern touches: men carrying banners in the processions suddenly falling out of line, running to lean their flags against the wall of the great Franciscan church before going off to shit their guts out; then, when the wards in the Umán IMSS clinic filled up, doctors and nurses putting IV drips on the people right where they had fallen.

Alejandro was called by the director of the T-1 and informed that he had been put in charge of the cholera effort. This, he notes, despite being under a cloud for the safer-sex information episode.

Cholera on top of SIDA: a plague on a plague. Russell's and Alejandro's regular patients wander in, wonder mildly where their doctors are, mention they've been waiting. Told about the emergency, they nod, understand, go off.

Alejandro thinks the Catholic Church should cancel all pilgrimages like the one to the Virgin of Umán at least until the cholera outbreak (which is all over southern Mexico and has been going on for several years) subsides. Or at least they should truck in safe water for the people to use during the festivities.

The diarrhea is so virulent that at the T-1 people are being placed on a kind of cloth stretcher with a hole in the middle and a container underneath. No use trying to get anyone up to make it to the bathroom, because you go thirty or forty times in a day. José Manuel's older sister, who is also a nurse here, comes in laughing about how all morning the elevators have been awash in the *sucia* of the poor people being brought in. "They have to keep bailing them out," she says. In Umán, so many folks are sick that they are being laid out crosswise, three to a bed.

The outbreak has the entire staff at the T-1 working overtime. Russell cancels his regular clinic hours for VIH-positive patients in order to minister to the stricken ("up there running around with his little water pitcher, saying, 'Can I get you a drink, señora?' just like Mother Teresa," is the report). The additional drama puts people in a good mood. There is little danger (though Alejandro does warn Elsa, their new part-time secretary, that it may be safer not to eat in the hospital cafeteria for a few days). A green-eyed young resident in surgery from the Chiapas border town of Comitán, whom we eat with at midday, reports how completely baffled he was when he arrived at the Juárez

Hospital this morning. "I couldn't find any of my patients. It turned out they had all been shuffled about to make more space for cholera." A lot of the cholera sufferers, the women especially, don't speak Spanish and become scared and disoriented. Many have never spent the night in a hospital before. In Umán, and here too, families wait around the clinic entrances trying to get news or pass a word in to their relatives. Because of the chaos and the contagiousness, visitors are not allowed upstairs. While we wait for our food, Alejandro, the nurses, and the resident trot out the Maya they know: "Sit down, please." "Open your mouth, please." "Show me your tongue." "Good." The nurses know more than the doctors.

The peninsula's hard limestone crust makes it difficult and time-consuming to dig latrine trenches. So in the villages people continue to defecate in vacant lots or the fields. In the rainy season the runoff carries the bacteria from the feces down into the underground water and people's backyard wells become infected.

The transmission route is human to human. The means of controlling cholera are simple and inexpensive. Boiling for twenty minutes renders water safe. Chlorinated water is cholera-free, and chlorine in concentrate disinfects surfaces where the bacteria may linger. Washing your hands with soap helps keep the infection from spreading. Chemical lime spread on human waste destroys the bacteria and keeps them from trickling down into the water supply.

By the end of the week the outbreak begins to subside. The hospitals have run out of serum and stretchers with the convenient hole in the center, and they have had to charter a plane to go pick up additional supplies in Veracruz. Saturday afternoon, when Alejandro and I return from a session of an IMSS conference called "Health and the Worker," a big truck is backed up to the front of the hospital and huge square plastic containers of chlorine are being unloaded.

The state government continues to deny that Umán has had five hundred cases of cholera. "Gastroenteritis," they say. *Novedades*, one of the more liberal dailies, reminds its readers that last year the government also refused to admit to a larger outbreak, six hundred cases in the Gulf town of Celestún. But the Mexico City papers carry the Umán story, so the nation and the world are aware of what the state government tries to cover up.

Why the denial? Because a continuing plague of cholera is one of the symbols not only of underdevelopment, but of a state apparatus that has neglected to provide even the simplest and most general health protections for its citizens. The *Novedades* reporter had talked with local leaders in some of the villages around Umán. They said they had been promised both chlorine and bags of lime by government officials, but none had arrived yet. Were they supposed to go to town to pick the stuff up? they asked. If so, the local people said, there is a problem, because *they* didn't even have the money to pay the *flete* (transportation).

Eighty-five percent of the ten thousand cases of SIDA reported in Mexico over the last ten years have been in men. But the percentage of cases in women has been rising, and now appears to have leveled off at about one in five of new cases, or 20 percent. Alejandro's figures for the southeast vary only slightly from the national pattern. In 1988 the female/male ratio here was one to thirteen; in 1991, one to five.

His estimate of the number of people in the region who are VIH-positive and who will become ill in the next decade is between 2,800 and 4,800. The estimate is based on seropositivity figures for three different groups: blood donors at IMSS, who can be thought of as representing a "general population" and who test positive at a *very* low rate (8 individuals out of 10,939 would-be donors in a one-year period); patients tested because of other, possibly VIH-related illnesses, 1.1 percent; and people with "risk practices," 7.9 percent (this group includes not only homosexual and bisexual men, but women who have been their partners).

Alejandro's projection is low (compared, for example, to Dr. Góngora-Biachi's assumption four years ago that there were 10,000 VIH-positive homosexual men in Mérida alone), but Alejandro's figures are in no way comforting. The three states of the *sureste* reported 284 cases in the first nine-and-a-half years of the SIDA epidemic. Alejandro's *low* estimate for the next ten years is ten times that.

Among patients at the T-1 last year, nineteen died of SIDA-related causes, a casualty every two-and-a-half weeks. People are living longer with VIH disease than they did before. The antiviral drugs appear to extend lives, treatment of opportunistic infections has become more sophisticated, expertise in the use of medications has grown. It also seems that both physicians and clients have come to recognize symptoms earlier in the course of the disease. However, all these improvements in the situation remain of more advantage to men than to women, who are still diagnosed later and whose average lifespan after diagnosis remains notably shorter than men's. Comparison of survival rates for patients who take AZT versus those who do not over the last three years make the drug appear *highly* effective. In the annual cohort of 1990, two-thirds of those on AZT survived (ten out of fifteen), while none of those who did not take the drug survived (zero out of ten). However, these comparisons do not take into account how far the disease has progressed in individual clients. The people who do not go on the antiviral are those who are very ill or near death at the time they are diagnosed.

Since 1990, SIDA has become the leading cause of death at the T-1 for both men and women between the ages of fifteen and fifty-four (supplanting the various sorts of cirrhosis—whether from alcohol use or local environmental factors). However, the sixteen SIDA deaths in 1990 represented less than 1 percent (0.89) of *total* deaths among IMSS clients for the year, and the nineteen in 1991 represented only 1.7 percent of deaths. In Mexico, as in the United States, from adolescence well into middle age, not many people die.

The fear AIDS generates must bear some relation to the fact that people die of it at a time in their lives when they have a reasonable expectation that they are not going to die. Early on, in the United States, the press pontificated about AIDS spreading because of a "godlike" refusal on the part of the [silly] homosexuals and the [callow or willfully ignorant] adolescents to believe they could actually die. Much of the "shame" people feel about AIDS clearly comes from its association with stigmatized sex and stigmatized sexuality. But people with AIDS may also feel guilty because they think now they will not be able to complete all the implicit contracts we make with one another—to provide for them or, more simply, to be present as friend or lover or parent for the long haul.

My lover went back to school and got his BA degree at the age of forty. Two months later he found out he was HIV-positive. He used to get drunk and cry and tell me the worst part of it was now he wouldn't be able to do what he had planned, which was to get a high-paying job and support me, since I had supported him for so many years. My father died of Hodgkin's disease when he was thirty-eight. I was only seven, but it became clear to me from the way the grown-ups talked that his death was not only "tragic," but also somehow horrible and unnatural because he was so young and was taking leave of his responsibilities to us at the wrong moment.

"Don Pablo" is a short, fifty-seven-year-old gentleman with silvery, receding hair and a $70 or $80 leather appointment book. Introduced during a pause while José Manuel is on the phone, he shakes hands with me and sits down rather carefully in the other chair at José Manuel's desk. Then, while he and José Manuel chat, I notice Don Pablo's legs are spread and his fingers are touching lightly along a big bulge on the left side of his crotch. Is he—mildly enough or even absentmindedly—showing himself off to me? But even as I wonder this, Don Pablo is saying no, he didn't drive, his car's in the shop again and he had to take the bus. "It was," he says, turning to include me, "an agony." His hand moves over to lie gently a moment over the whole lump, which is the size of a mature mango. "Even getting this thing up the stairs onto the bus hurts. Not to mention there is *no* comfortable way I can sit anymore."

"What is it?" I ask.

Don Pablo shrugs and sighs. "Who knows? *They* don't know. A tumor maybe. Sometimes they say it may be a granuloma."

He is here today to get an appointment with a surgeon. Russell and Alejandro want to try to drain the growth with a needle to see if that gives him some relief. To stand, Don Pablo supports himself first, both fists pushing down on the surface of José Manuel's desk, then lifts his torso up. Once he's on his feet, the lump is not obvious in his slacks.

José Manuel asks, "How are you going to get home, Don Pablo?"

"Oh, they're coming to pick me up. It's all right."

By chance, the next visitor is Inés, the softer of the two transvestites who came for their VIH test while I was here in March. Today, her brown hair is down around her shoulders and she has on a short black-and-white checkered skirt, stockings, heels, and a white blouse with a swooping, frilled V-neck which provides a little peek of a lacy bra. Inés's test result is again negative. She barely looks at the slip of paper José Manuel gives her before tucking it into her purse. He starts to introduce me, but Inés says of course she remembers me. She holds out her hand and we shake, then she thanks both José Manuel and me profusely and gives Alejandro a big smile on her way out. Ten minutes later I give my hand to José Manuel to sniff. It still smells strongly of Inés's nice gardenia-scented cologne.

Don Pablo returns and again carefully takes a seat. The surgeon they wanted him to see doesn't have an opening for two weeks, so Don Pablo settles for coming back tomorrow without an appointment to see Russell.

He admits to José Manuel that he sometimes forgets to take his medication, especially his AZT. José Manuel tells him, "In the morning when you first get up, make everything you're supposed to take that day up into little packets and write the time on the outside. Then, at ten o'clock or noon or whenever you're supposed to have them, no matter where you are, your pills will be there in your pocket and you can just take them. That way you don't have to carry the bottles around with you or anything."

Don Pablo keeps his IMSS card stuck in the front of his leather appointment book. Across from it, under plastic, is a snapshot of a lean, chesty young man in a scant bathing suit, the beach white behind him.

I am alone in the office when three people come in, more or less at the same moment, looking for José Manuel. A family, I assume. The boy, who has on a T-shirt, sprawls across from me at the round table and leans his forehead on his hand. Father, a heavy-boned, cavernous, scowling six-footer with short, mossy dark hair, and Mother, a tiny, jerky, lightweight bird with hair so thin and straggly you can tell the precise shape of her head, sit straight and silent at José Manuel's desk. Intense, poisonous silence resonates between the generations, which causes me to imagine that Dad and Mom must have caught Sonny here at something sexual (whether with another boy or with a girl I can't tell) and as part of a course in warning and humiliation have brought him in for testing.

José Manuel returns and tells the adults he's going to deal with the young man first and will be with them in a moment. It turns out that they are not related at all. The boy is here only to learn his test result, which is negative. When he leaves, José Manuel has the couple move over to the typing table so he can complete the paperwork for the man to get his stipend and lab orders for the trip to Mexico City for the T cell test.

While José Manuel hammers away at the typewriter, the couple begin to fill me in on details. He only found out two weeks ago, the man says. He became suspicious because he'd lost a lot of weight, more than 25 pounds (13 kilos) and though he's a diabetic, he didn't think that was the cause. Recently, he says, he's become very emotional. His wife nods abruptly. "Wakes up in the middle of the night crying," she says.

José Manuel refers to the man's chart. "The medication Dr. Russell has put you on should help calm you down. But beyond that, the best medicine for your nerves would be for you to spend more time reading, or at quiet things, and to worry less, begin to live your life now to the fullest and not to spend a lot of time alone having bad thoughts."

The man wants to know if instead of going to the D.F. on the bus he could apply the travel stipend toward an airplane ticket. José Manuel tells him yes, he can. A minute later, looking over one of the forms he has to carry with him, the man mentions that all this is going to cost IMSS a lot. "Well," says José Manuel, "remember, that's what you've been paying your money in for all these years. In exchange, you get the best treatment we can possibly give you."

The couple are still around the T-1 well into the afternoon. I come on them sometimes together, or her by herself, waiting outside an office, sitting on the stone wall of the courtyard in the shade while her husband is getting his documents signed and stamped. At one point when he and I are alone, he tells me that he has been a manager at another clinic for thirty years, has spent his life around doctors. He became infected from going to prostitutes, he says.

It's not just imagining that Don Pablo was groping himself when he wasn't, or thinking that the clinic manager and his wife were the parents of the surly boy. I continue to discover that I missed a lot of things when I was here five months ago. I recognize that slippage—misunderstanding—is a part of ordinary life, that it happens on home territory, and that in another culture, another language, it is bound to happen even more. It becomes, actually, the major way an outsider learns. But still, I find the little mistakes embarrass me, make me doubt myself as a reporter, remind me we always proceed, make our decisions, large and small, on partial (and partly bad) information.

The bigger misapprehensions also trouble me, but I have a better understanding of how they came about, what in the way I perceive things led me to draw a certain conclusion. For example, Hugo Vargas, the attractive young *promotor* who showed up one day at the clinic and hung around, the one whose quiet style I thought would make him an excellent SIDA outreach worker: "What happened with him?" I ask José Manuel. "Do you ever see him?"

"No, we don't. You know, Carter, it turned out that Hugo is a little crazy. He's an epileptic and he takes a lot of drugs for it. Maybe that's what makes him so *fofo*."

"*Fofo*? What does that mean?"

"You remember, how Hugo was, so sweet and soft."

"And what's the form of his craziness?"

"It seems he goes around letting people believe he's a doctor. Things like that."

I was not trained in statistics, which means that I end up going back to Alejandro over and over again for explanations of his tables.

I understand his estimate of new cases of SIDA in the peninsula for the next ten years is based on projections from the incidence of seropositivity in different groups tested for VIH at IMSS. But how can a projection be developed for the "at risk" group (homosexual and bisexual men and their women partners) when no one really knows how large it is? Four years ago, Dr. Góngora-Biachi and his colleagues used the census figure of forty thousand unmarried male heads of household over thirty as their guess for the number of adult male homosexuals in Mérida (and, as mentioned earlier, then projected 25 percent of these, or ten thousand men, as already seropositive). But even if the single male head of household figure was correct, who has an accurate figure on the number of male bisexuals either in the city or in the entire peninsula?

The other problem with Alejandro's estimate is that I don't think it accounts for a possible *acceleration* in the seropositivity rates among various groups. And, of course, if education about how to protect yourself from infection is not more effective in the second decade of SIDA in the *sureste* than it was in the first, the *rate* of infection will certainly increase as surely as will the number of people who become ill.

Alejandro's low estimate of the cumulative number of cases for the second decade of SIDA is ten times that for the first, his high estimate is more than sixteen times. Whatever their faults, his projections would be useful to anyone trying to plan what the medical system will need in the near future in order to deal with the disease. The current patient load at the T-1 requires the major portion of the effort of two infectious disease specialists and one full-time nurse and regularly occupies three or four hospital beds. But the staff and the number of beds needed by the year 2002 will be *more* than ten times the current level, given the acceleration in the number of cases to be expected as the decade proceeds. Of course, the fact is that no one is actually *planning* for SIDA in the next ten years.

Four years ago Renán Góngora outlined for me a possible route for the spread of SIDA into Mayan communities, but said the risk of the disease actually spreading widely to the countryside was "minimal." The news from Wakax indicates how wise his thinking was about a route of transmission, and how wrong about the chance SIDA would "jump" to the villages.

José Manuel repeats to his friends Niko and Stella that in the office I am like his and Alejandro's shadow. Though I don't think he is being critical, I do begin to feel in the way. Alejandro is aware that I'm supposed to be skilled in figuring out how things go in traditional life. When am I going to start using those skills? Yesterday he mentioned the street corner where I could catch the bus that goes out to Wakax. Last night I had trouble sleeping, thinking about the town, wondering where I might sling a hammock there, what I could accomplish. In the end I knew there was really no decision to make right now. I go back to California to teach in less than a week, and there is no use trying to set up shop in Wakax or any other Mayan town in such a short time. Still, lying there in the dark, sweating away despite the heavy drone of the hotel air conditioner, I couldn't help framing everything in terms of my lack of courage in a crisis.

A man and a woman come into the office, both of them thin and small, she in little clear plastic slipperlike shoes with silver glitter caught in the plastic, he in a faded black T-shirt and dusty baseball cap. They are Nestor and Alicia, the married clients from Wakax. José Manuel sits Alicia down across from him at the typing desk, Nestor stands to the side and slightly behind her with his arms folded over his chest.

José Manuel tells them they need to get to know other people facing the same problems they have. He says to Alicia, "It's especially important for you, señora, to meet other women in the same situation, because—"

Before he can finish, she lowers her head and begins to weep.

José Manuel says, "Don't cry, señora."

Alejandro has been at something else at his own desk. Now he comes over and explains that the people at this organization called Ya'ax Che are going to try to help Nestor and Alicia with the money for the bus to Mexico City. Alicia takes a little handkerchief from her pocket and wipes at her face. José Manuel gives them directions on how to get from the Zócalo to the Association and writes out the address, which he hands to Nestor.

After they leave, José Manuel catches Alejandro's eye and shakes his head. Alejandro tells me, "They have *got* to go there, you know. And not only for the group meetings. Georgina can give them the nutritional supplements, too. Protein. You can see they both need that already."

Nestor has confided to Alejandro that he's been getting terrible headaches. They come from thinking, he says, about how unhappy he has made his wife, all through their marriage, getting drunk and beating her (in this it was a "Mexican marriage," Alejandro says), and from thinking how now he's given her this terrible disease and there is no way to make it up to her.

They were married young, Alicia only fifteen or sixteen at the time.

Friday morning early, 7:15 A.M., a tiny balding gentleman, his thinning hair carefully combed back, gray at the temples, stands before José Manuel's desk in a pressed fresh Dacron *guayabera*. His son, he explains, now has the trembles and shakes, and the nurses upstairs have informed them this is about the end. "What we need to know, then, is what we need to do. Will we have to report to anyone? What about clothes?"

José Manuel says, "The doctors will make the report. You shouldn't worry about that. All you will need to do is bring in what you want the nurses to put on him." The little gentleman nods. "And remember it remains your choice," José Manuel says, "whether you want to bury Héctor or have him cremated."

The father nods and says, "We are aware of everything."

For the English-speaker—in Spanglais—the way the little gentleman put it sounded vast, encompassing: "*Estámos consciente de todo.*" Later, after the weekend, Russell took me with him up to the third floor and into a small room on the opposite side of the hall from the wards. The shade was drawn, and gathered around the bed in the gloom were Héctor's father, his mother, and my friend from the Asociación Ya'ax Che, José Luis Matú, who had on a wide black sleeveless top, a crucifix, and several other pendants around his neck and (my memory insists) his black porkpie hat. The boy on the bed was emaciated, awake, his eyes huge, a startled look. Russell asked him how he was doing, but Héctor just continued to stare. "Ah, I see," Russell said. On the way back downstairs, he told me the father runs a cantina, and Héctor got started having sex with men as a kid working in his father's place as a waiter. His parents have agreed to let Héctor be autopsied. It will be the first time at the T-1 that a postmortem will be performed on a patient who has died of SIDA complications.

Before eight o'clock, two boys arrive for their alpha interferon injections. One of them, Salem, a Lebanese with precise features, is just beginning the treatment, and José Manuel takes the time to ask if someone at home can give him his shots on the weekend.

"Yes, my sister does injections," says Salem. "But during the week I'd rather come and have you do it, if that's all right."

José Manuel says, "That's what I'd prefer too. That way I'll finally get you alone with your pants down. The shot goes under the skin, not into the muscle or a vein, and we use a rotation method, right arm, left arm, left thigh, right thigh"—showing the places on himself as he names them—"so we'll always know where we've hit last."

"Does it hurt?"

"Not that much."

The little flat boxes, each containing the two vials that need to be mixed for one treatment, are entrusted to the clients, together with disposable syringes and needles. Salem peels his shirt back from his shoulders. José Manuel injects him and then tosses the needle into the ordinary, lidless cardboard box in the corner where he is currently putting all of his used needles, bandages, and swabs. Salem moves his shoulders a bit, then shrugs, pulls his shirt back over his shoulders and rebuttons it.

Tomorrow José Manuel will be thirty-two. At midmorning, a skinny client in his fifties, a man with big ears, quick motions, and a persistent cough, is sitting with José Manuel. He holds a black plastic bag. The man has just been released from the hospital, and they are talking about how soon he can make the trip to Mexico City for the T helper test. "Whenever you get your strength back," José Manuel tells him. They agree on ten days or two weeks. Getting up to go, the man sneaks from his plastic bag a flat box wrapped in gold paper. "Here," he says, "I heard it was your birthday, José Manuel."

José Manuel thanks the client, but does not open the present while he is in the room. Just as the client is leaving, Elsa, the new typist, comes in. She is followed by a shuffling sandy-haired fellow named Andrés, who has a tote bag over his shoulder. Andrés wears a raggedy T-shirt and a visored black sailor's cap. He has prominent, irregular teeth and thick glasses, a grown-up child in his thirties. José Manuel and Elsa speculate about what the birthday present might be. From its shape they guess a pen-and-pencil set. But when he unwraps the box, it turns out to be a gold-plated ID bracelet with José Manuel's name engraved on it. Though José Manuel is already wearing one gold bracelet, he adds the new one to his wrist and shows it off to one and all. Drawing near for a look, Andrés announces that he, too, had heard it was José Manuel's birthday and has something for him. From the tote bag come two boxes, both wrapped in tatty flowered paper with crushed and battered bows, all held together with plenty of Scotch tape. José Manuel is so busy admiring his new gold bracelet that he hardly remembers to thank Andrés for what he has brought.

But once Andrés leaves, José Manuel tears open the new boxes. In one is a bar of perfumed soap from Revlon's "Charlie" line, pushed some years ago in the States with Lauren Hutton as its sales icon; in the other is a round plastic container of "Charlie" face powder with a powder puff inside. In her twenty-three-year-old's openness of heart, Elsa goes "Oooh," but neither José Manuel or I say anything. When he puts the lid back on, a little explosion of the finest white dust blows out in all directions across the table. José Manuel sits at Elsa's desk and tries for a moment to contain himself, taking deep hoarse breaths—huff, huff, harumph—and then begins to cry.

At about one o'clock Elsa brings in his birthday cake, a very large pink-icing affair that she has arranged. Eight or nine people gather at the round table for a slice. I sit next to Jenny, whom I have not seen before on this trip. She had her baby, a boy, in the middle of July, she tells me, and is very happy. This is her first week back at work. They had to do a cesarean section, she says, lightly drawing the line across her stomach to indicate the cut. Jenny works away at the extra big piece of cake they have given her, but in the end it's too much for her, so she puts a second paper plate on top of it and takes the rest away to eat later.

José Manuel is out of the office when a young man named Miguel Ángel comes to deliver *his* neatly wrapped offering. Up-to-the-minute stylish in his black pants and white dress shirt, narrow black suspenders and white loafers, Miguel Ángel remembers me from Russell's clinic last March. He is an office assistant in the administration section of the T-1, and at the moment his problem is an internal growth of some sort that has grossly distended the right side of his jaw. It unbalances and pulls Miguel Ángel's face, making him look like a not particularly happy cartoon character. Popeye, maybe. His polite, refined, quiet style does not at all jibe with the huge distortion of his face.

"Does it hurt?" I ask.

"It hasn't," he says, "but now it's beginning to."

"Is any of the infection in your mouth?"

"No. They think perhaps it's a lymphoma, but they don't know for sure yet."

What makes him feel awful, Miguel Ángel says, is that as part of his job he prepares coffee for his boss's guests, and he is ashamed to go into his boss's office looking the way he does. Specialists are supposed to examine the growth next week. Miguel Ángel promises to come tell me what they say.

After work, José Manuel and I splash across town in his car through huge puddles left by this afternoon's downpour, on our way to the Colonia Itzimná. Stopped at a red light, José Manuel recognizes the occupants of the Volkswagen bug next to us. The driver is a redheaded woman in a nurse's uniform, José Manuel's old friend Niko; her passenger is Stella, Niko's smoky blond girlfriend. Calling back and forth:

"Where are you going?"

"To have a beer."

"We are too. It's my birthday, come with us!"

"Where?"

"Eládio's—follow me!"

We park on a side street under the shade of wet trees and next to a wrought-iron fence. Through the bars are wide green lawns surrounding a lonely, closed-up mansion from the last century. On the sidewalk we step around a decaying, foul-smelling animal carcass, a huge rat I think at first, though it turns out to be an opossum.

Eládio's is a popular bar-restaurant (there are two other branches in Mérida) housed under a vast thatched roof. It is crowded today, and noisy. In order to talk, we take a table in a glassed-in, air-conditioned room in the back of the building. We begin with beer and consume large amounts of the delicious *botana*, which the waiters bring by on trays; the hard-egg tacos with ground pumpkinseed sauce, called *papadzules*; chicken with red *achiote* baked in banana leaves (*pollo pibil*); the hard, hot sausage called *longaniza*. After a while we move to *hiboles*, José Manuel and I to rum with Coke or mineral water, Stella to shots of tequila with glasses of soda as chasers, and Niko to shots of vodka drunk solo. Niko continually reorders the table, mopping up little spills with paper napkins, plopping more ice into the glasses.

She has been working extra hours on the second floor of the T-1, tending the people with cholera. But her regular shifts are on the third floor, and she knows all of the SIDA patients. We talk about Héctor, the son of the cantina owner who came in so early this morning to get José Manuel's instructions. Niko doesn't like the idea that arrangements have already been made to perform an autopsy when the poor guy hasn't even died yet. It's too spooky, she says, as though you were *wishing* the person gone.

Apparently it is optional for the nurses to do the washing and first laying out of the dead. A friend of Niko's mother passed away, "a woman I knew from my earliest childhood on," she says. Niko had tended the old lady all the way through, and they were there in the hall, she and the daughter, crying and holding each other in their arms, when Niko saw the other nurses about to go into the woman's room. "And I told them, 'No, here, give *me* that stuff, that's *my* duty you know,' and I went in to her myself. It was the last thing I was able to do for my mother's friend, and for my friend too, and for the family. In the end it's not so much a duty, really, as an honor to be able to do that for someone."

Later, Stella tells us she has a really bad stomach and this drinking is killing her. But she continues, she says with a laugh, she perseveres.

And as we talk on, she consumes plate after plate of the *longaniza*. Her parents—her mother especially—get on her for staying out drinking, not coming home at night. But she doesn't care, she says, tossing her curls, looking possessively across to Niko.

The rain returns, drumming heavily on the tin roof that covers this part of the building. The band has finished for the evening, and Eládio's has begun to clear out. Niko and Stella speak with some fondness about how they fight, but how they care for each other, too. It's complicated for her, Niko says, because she's the older. She's been married and had her dear son. "And then," brightly, as though it was magic when it happened, "*this* child—," she says, meaning Stella. But she can't complete the thought. Niko shrugs, drinks. "I am myself," she says, "I do what I do, that's all."

Niko is showing off a gold-plated ring, which is the graduation souvenir from a particular additional certification course she took through one of the hospitals, when suddenly José Manuel bursts into tears. She puts her hand on his forearm, shakes him. "José Manuel? What's wrong with you?"

"I was going to take that specialty, before they threw me out of there—"

"Oh, *chulo*—"

"But now that I know I'm going to die—"

Both women are on their feet, leaning over José Manuel, hugging him. Niko puts her chin to his forehead and strokes his hair. "You're *not* going to die," she tells him, "you're not."

José Manuel calms down. Almost as suddenly as it lapsed, his good humor reappears and, though still weeping, he is telling the women the story of this morning's gold bracelet, followed by the gifts from Andrés: "The old gentleman is a thousand times richer than that poor kid—but Andrés's packages, the way they were with their ends and their tape sticking out all over, the two of them coming together like that, it made me realize that our clients *do* understand what my work is all about, and that made me cry."

It is nine o'clock before we leave Eládio's. José Manuel has become amorous, stroking my leg under the table, asking if it's all right if he comes back to the hotel with me, licking his fingers while the waiter stands by and Niko, Stella, and I regard the bill. I contribute what I have, about U.S. $60, and the women put in the rest, which is about $30. The rain has finally stopped, but outside, by our cars, the trees shed big cold raindrops onto us as we all four embrace. Then José Manuel and I are tooling in town along the Montejo, radio blaring, kissing, hands on each other, steaming up the windshield. "If we don't calm down, I'm going to crash into something," he tells me. And a minute later, he bucks into a pothole and flattens a tire. Prophesy fulfilled. He steers the car, limping on the rim, onto a side street, and José Manuel, who has no jack, goes off to call Jorge Solís to come rescue us. By the time Jorge arrives, a half-hour later, other friends have also stopped to see if they can help, and both José Manuel and I have sobered up some. Jorge and I get someone else's jack to work, and José Manuel loses interest in the tire problem. "We'll just let the men do it," he tells the others with a wave in our direction.

They say the rain should have ended in August, but the dramatic thunderstorms continue almost every afternoon or in the early evening. My hotel room this time is on the sixth floor facing north. The dark clouds ride in quickly, racing across the peninsula from the east off the Atlantic, vast flights of birds running before them. Out across the flat green city, marked by the radio towers and the high-rise hotels, you can see block by block where the storm has already begun. There is wind, and along the horizon thick bolts of electricity connect sky to earth. Then the boom of the thunder and the clattering rain, steaming when it first hits the hot pavement, and, in the premature dark, the mercury lamps in the park a block down glow and then come on. Soon the streets are full of flowing, grayish, opaque water, lapping onto the sidewalks when a bus plows by. A little old lady in a *huipil* drapes her arms around her grandson's neck and lets him carry her through the flood. When the storm ends, or settles into a more constant rain, the city is just as hot as it was before.

It rained Thursday night for the opening of the IMSS conference on health and the worker, which was held in a seventh-floor meeting room of one of the tourist hotels on the Montejo. I arrived a bit late and wet and stood at the back with several doctors I recognized from the T-1. Up front, behind the flower-decked table where the dignitaries sat, a kind of set had been constructed for the event, panels of white on which big green styrofoam letters spelled out IMSS and the name of the conference and the IMSS logo. Several handsome young women, looking like airline stewardesses in their green and white *Seguro* outfits, were there to offer general assistance and to serve, it appeared, as decoration.

At the last minute, the organizers of the conference had asked Alejandro to be master of ceremonies at the opening session. After some hesitation, he agreed. This in addition to being put in charge of the cholera effort and being asked to consider taking charge of problems concerning infectious disease *across* the various hospitals in Mérida. I asked him if he thought they were pushing him *up* as a way of neutralizing him on the question of SIDA. "It's strange, isn't it?" Alejandro said. "Last week the director of Public Health telling me I was unruly, lacking discipline, and now all this."

He was standing now by the podium in his best *guayabera*, eyes on the ceiling, as the federal delegates and the IMSS *jefes* from Mexico City welcomed one another. Instead of passing the microphone back to Alejandro so he could make the introductions, the politicos simply passed it around among themselves. In their remarks they left no cliché unturned, including mention of "our Yucatán" as the "land of the pheasant and the deer." The governor was supposed to appear, but she did not show up, so after about three-quarters of an hour the honored guests and the fifty or so tired doctors and their coiffed wives got up from their folding chairs and bowed their heads, and the chief delegate delivered a brief invocation and declared the conference open. Pause. Applause. A rite of self-worship (no god invoked) on the part of the state bureaucracy. Then a short break while the politicos made their way out of the room, shaking hands and putting their arms around a number of people's shoulders.

Saturday morning at 10:00, Alejandro has a session on SIDA in the same room, for which I arrive on time. Unfortunately, the main speaker from the previous colloquium on planning is just being introduced. He is a good-looking fellow about forty, a high-level bureaucrat in a spanking white *guayabera*. For a while everyone tries to listen to his prepared speech on "models for correct decision making." When the room goes dark for his overhead projections, people shift in their seats and try to rouse themselves. But the "visuals" turn out to be complicated organizational flow charts with lots of thick arrows, and for some reason turning the lights down *increases* the already dense buzzing of the room's air conditioning. Some people go off to try to reduce the sound, as the diagrams begin to remind me of basement passageways of great old big-city hotels with their mazes of overhead pipes and heating ducts. The problem with the speaker's "model" for "democratic process" is that it has nothing to do with hard decisions made for reasons of money.

In Alejandro's session the audience becomes alert. It is, after all, their colleagues who are speaking. The psychiatrist from the T-1 they call "Doctor David" lists the stages of the VIH-positive person "coming to terms" with the disease: depression, questioning "why me?", eventual resignation, and then acceptance. The dermatologist shows lurid slides, mouths full of candidiasis, a raw outbreak of herpes simplex snaking up out of the crack of somebody's buttocks, more delicate discolorations on a patient's face which are, in fact, lesions of Karposi's Sarcoma. Alejandro's speech is about the senselessness of trying to require people to take VIH tests as a condition of employment. He quotes the World Health Organization's position against such requirements and talks about the importance of helping affected people to continue as long as possible as producers, economically useful and self-supporting. After the session, cookies and coffee are served, and the presenters and their friends go about complimenting one another. Unlike some of their colleagues, these doctors all seem to conceive SIDA as a set of problems with which they must familiarize themselves.

Later, Alejandro tells me the top administrator from the D.F. who was at the conference buttonholed him and said *his* current biggest problem was that at the IMSS hospitals in the capital there were a lot of doctors who were clearly *putos*, and who also clearly had the disease. But they didn't want to retire. How, he asked Alejandro, was he going to get them out?

Saturday afternoon we are back at the T-1 where things are very quiet. Alejandro goes upstairs to look in on the cholera patients and is gone a long time. When he returns, we go across the street to have a beer. Upstairs, Alejandro tells me, he ran into the doctor who had reported him to the Public Health director over the safer-sex mimeograph. Now, suddenly, this doctor is changing his tune, saying he thinks what Alejandro needs is additional staff, a social worker, a psychologist, a full-time secretary. And a more "confidential" clinic, with more space so they can have their own little waiting room, away from the one for the general public.

Monday. I ask Alejandro how yesterday went for him (we were both out Saturday until 4:00 A.M. in further celebration of José Manuel's birthday). He says he tried to get some sleep, but the family of one of his patients came to find him. The man is dying at home, and has been unconscious for several days now. Though he was diagnosed several months ago, the patient, a married man, has refused all treatment and held off telling his family what was wrong with him as long as he possibly could. He signed a document requesting that *no* medical effort be made for him at any point, so even though he is unconscious, it is permissible that his family not bring him into the hospital. Sunday the family asked if it were possible to give him something to help him die, but Alejandro had to tell them that he wasn't permitted to provide such things.

A woman comes in with her son. She now lives in Tuxtla Gutiérrez, the state capital of Chiapas, and is back only for a visit. Her boy, Lázaro, is seven, clear white milky skin and big eyes, a hemophiliac, VIH-positive. Lázaro has an older brother who is also a hemophiliac, but not VIH-positive. While Alejandro and the mother talk, José Manuel calls the boy over. "Lázaro, you didn't even say hello to me." Lázaro plays with José Manuel's round rack of official stamps, stamping various pieces of paper and the back of his own and José Manuel's hands in purple ink. The earpieces of Lázaro's plastic sunglasses are broken. José Manuel tries to rig something up using string, but the experiment is a failure.

Alejandro has a letter about Lázaro for the woman to take back with her to the doctors in Tuxtla, an assessment, meant to alert them to changes in the boy's health they need to be on the lookout for. A case like Lázaro's is very specialized, and not everyone would be trained to know how to deal with it. He's not taking AZT at the moment. Alejandro points out to the mother how well he's doing, how healthy he looks, but she rejects this idea. "Look how thin he is. He won't put on any weight. I'm afraid to let him play with anyone, even his own brothers," she says.

She knew Alejandro when he and the mother of his little boy were still together, so she is surprised and sorry to learn they have split up.

Alejandro tells her about the engineer his wife met, and how they are going to live together in another part of the country.

"But how can they do that? What about your little boy?"

"They're leaving this week, in fact."

"But how? He's your son, too."

"Well, that's the way it is," Alejandro says. "She came to ask me to sign the paper and I signed it."

The woman is about to go, but then she comes back and leans over Alejandro's desk. "What about a vaccine? I listen all the time to the television and I try to stay informed, but it's hard to find that kind of news."

"No," Alejandro says, "no vaccine yet. Maybe in time."

Later in the week, on short notice, Alejandro and I decide to take an overnight trip down through Quintana Roo to the lake of Bacalar and the city of Chetumal. On the way back we can visit some of the places still occupied by the Cruzob, the living descendants of the Mayan rebels of the War of the Castes in the last century. After the Puuc Hills and Ticul it will be all new territory for me, but for Alejandro the road is familiar, since he worked in Chetumal as a young man, and Chunhuhub, which is along the way, is where his oldest son was born. As we are leaving Mérida Saturday afternoon, Alejandro tells me he dreamed last night that he was visiting all the different houses his parents had rented in the D.F. when he and his brothers and sisters were kids, but the houses were all packed up, ready to move.

I ask did they live in a lot of different places when he was growing up. Alejandro says not so many, four or five maybe.

"Will you get to see your son before they leave?"

"They've already gone. She left yesterday," Alejandro says.

I sit talking with Laura, the tall, blond woman who became VIH-positive through a blood transfusion when she had plastic surgery on her nose. She talks about *her* son, almost four now, she says, and completely mischievous and into trouble. And smart and wonderful. He doesn't want to go to school—"Nobody there loves me the way you do, Mama," he says—and when he has to go, he gets in fights.

Laura's own family is in Morelia. She has no one here. Her husband rejects her, and the people in his family tell her, "Why don't you just get out of the way?" Alejandro tells her she would be better off going back to her own family, who are supportive of her. But she says she can't, because of the boy.

The husband has plenty of money. He's spent it on a new house, on other girlfriends. Mental abuse, Alejandro says. The *pattern* is a typical one in Mexico. Articles have been written about it. Men who are VIH-negative reject their wives when they test positive, don't trust them. Even when there's clear proof the women were infected by some other means, the husbands assume it was through a liaison with another man.

For a long time, Laura's only symptoms were colds that she found difficult to shake. Now, she has had thrush in her mouth for three months. The medication Alejandro thinks will take care of it is expensive and is not one that IMSS gives out, but Laura's husband refuses to give her the money to buy it.

There is a knock at the office door and I let in a group of three: a skinny dark boy, a broad-faced older man with a bulbous nose, and a girl of fifteen or sixteen with lipstick, earrings, sandals. At first I think the older man is the driver who has brought the young couple in from Wakax. He has on a bright print shirt, green jungle leaves, orange and white fruit. But in fact he is the father of the boy, whose name is Bernardo, and who is seventeen.

All three sit around José Manuel's desk. José Manuel bustles across the room to retrieve a piece of paper, returns, and settles into his chair.

Bernardo introduces the girl as his *novia*.

"Are you married yet?" José Manuel asks.

"No."

José Manuel asks the girl, "Are you pregnant?"

"No."

José Manuel takes a deep breath. "Bernardo, would you like to talk alone with me or with the others present? Or we could be alone at first and then talk all together."

Bernardo thinks about it. He seems unable to make a decision.

"Then we'll go ahead all together?" José Manuel asks.

The tiniest nod from Bernardo.

"What I have to tell you, then, is something very serious," José Manuel says. "The result of your test was positive. What does it mean? That you have the virus for SIDA in your body. It does not mean that you are necessarily going to die of this particular thing, but it *does* mean your health is now going to become a very serious concern for you, Bernardo, and for us as well. We will want to test your *novia* today, and then we'll ask both of you to come back—" José Manuel thinks, Tuesday and Wednesday the T-1 is closed for the national holidays celebrating independence, "—on Thursday to get the result. From now on, neither of you should have sex with anyone but each other, and then only when you use a condom. The señorita won't want to get pregnant now. Do you understand me so far?" All nod. "When you come back Thursday we'll talk further about what to do for your health, Bernardo, how you can begin to improve your nutrition, eat better, more fish, more meat. Do you have a job?"

"No."

"So you're not registered in the IMSS system."

"No."

A big sigh from José Manuel. "Well, we'll still see what we can do."

José Manuel brings the girl over to the round table, sits her down, draws blood from her arm, leaves her the cotton swab to press against the puncture.

Her dress is a plum color, very good looking on her.

Though no one cries, everyone is solemn. After the girl's test, the father begins to ask angry questions. Who's responsible for all this? How did it come about?

"We don't know those things," José Manuel says. "And what we want to concentrate on right now is how we can do the best we possibly can for the young people, isn't it?"

The father is reluctant. "Well, yes."

It is not yet nine o'clock in the morning. Bernardo is the seventh VIH-bearer from Wakax. If his fiancée is seropositive, she will be number eight.

Later, Nestor and Alicia come in. They weren't able to find the Association Friday, so Alejandro gives them new directions and off they go again. Around two in the afternoon, they come back a second time. Alicia sits, Nestor stands behind her. The funds for their trip to Mexico City have still not been found. What if they took the train, which is cheaper than the bus? No, José Manuel tells them, that's no good. The only remaining through train takes three days each way. Alicia has on the same dress and the same clear plastic shoes with spangles in them she was wearing the other day. One more question, they say. But just then José Manuel gets a phone call from an "engineer" who wants to take him to lunch on Wednesday. His conversation goes on and on, and finally Alicia and Nestor walk over to Alejandro's desk to ask if *he* can help them. The problem is that now Alicia is having headaches, too. She thinks they must come from nerves. Could the doctor prescribe something for them?

Thursday morning, Bernardo, his father, and Bernardo's *novia* return. José Manuel is out today, so Alejandro rummages through the papers on his assistant's desk and finds the most recent test results. The girl's test is negative. The father nods and Bernardo sneaks a sideward glance of pleasure at her. Her back is to me, so I can't see her expression.

In the afternoon, Nestor comes in alone. José Manuel was supposed to help him write a petition in his own words to the governor to beg for the funds he and his wife need to get to Mexico City. But José Manuel still hasn't shown up, so Alejandro makes a call to a lawyer, then writes a note for Nestor to hand-deliver to the lawyer, who has agreed to help the couple. In the note Alejandro calls Nestor's and Alicia's dilemma a "situation of maximum anguish."

The phone rings while Nestor is waiting, and I answer it. It's José Manuel. Things must have gone well with your engineer, I say. Too well, he says, with a little laugh. He asks to speak to Alejandro.

Nestor continues to stand in front of José Manuel's desk. Both of us pretend not to listen to what Alejandro is saying. "I don't care if you miss a day from time to time, but at least *tell* me it's going to happen so I can get somebody else in here to do your job, or at least call me in the morning and let me know. You have duties to clients, too, you know. All the boys you give Intrón A injections to came this morning, but you weren't here so they all had to make other arrangements—" Nestor and I exchange a look, and a shy smile passes between us, that pleasure you get as a child when some other kid is being punished and for once it's not you.

The next morning another young man comes to the clinic at the T-1 to pick up his result. He is twenty-two, tall, with a spiky, gel-wet professional haircut, fashionably bleached jeans. Self-possessed, casual, at ease. He has lived in Los Angeles and now works as a waiter in Cancún, but in fact he is from Wakax, too. When Alejandro tells him he is positive for VIH, he simply nods, as though he knew all along. Number eight. He has questions, about what medicines are available, how long and how well a person can live with this thing. He has a girlfriend, he says, but they aren't married. He'll bring her in to take the test next week. He also volunteers to go around to boys and men he thinks could have had sex with the restaurant owner who died or with the two schoolteachers, to try to get them to come in and be tested as well.

Alejandro and I are both struck by how different this young man's reaction is from that of the others who came in from Wakax, the way he immediately began to look ahead, toward whatever life might still have for him. Yet he arouses something else in us, too. Despite his time in the States and his sophistication about the disease, he is, as Alejandro puts it, "living proof that the educational programs aren't working."

José Manuel, who drew the blood, says that this young man told him he had had a bad case of syphilis in Los Angeles a couple of years ago. "So instead of being infected in the village, maybe he got the virus up there—where all these things come from," says José Manuel.

The man I met in March who travels for the medical supply company is in for a checkup. While he is with Russell, his wife drops in to see José Manuel.

"How are we doing? Well *he's* fine, as far as I can tell. I'm the one who's nervous. Can't sleep at night. Dr. Russell tells me I should *read*, but I know what the real therapy for me would be—"

"I do too, *chula*—"

"José Manuel!" She reaches across and playfully slaps his hand. "No, what I really need is something *you* could provide, my dear. To go out and spend the whole night dancing."

"Well, we'll do it then."

A few minutes later when her husband and Russell come in, she tells them it's all set, she's going to get *her* "therapy" from José Manuel. Everyone laughs.

Then she and I are both sitting at José Manuel's desk, and she tells us confidentially, "There's nothing wrong with *him*, you know. It's me. I know it's supposed to be all right, completely safe, but in bed—afterward?—he goes right off to sleep, but I just lie there and lie there and I can't sleep at all the rest of the night. Isn't that foolish?"

"No, señora," we both say, "not foolish at all."

Andrés, the boy who brought José Manuel the soap and the "Charlie" face powder, comes shuffling in and methodically takes photographs from his ever-present tote bag to show anyone who will have a look at them. There are pictures of Andrés as a fairly normal-appearing schoolboy, and snapshots of family members. One larger school group photo is in a stand-up plastic frame in the shape of Mickey Mouse's dog Pluto. Trying to find something polite to ask Andrés, I pick a tattered black and white picture of what appears to be a gnomish little old man in a doorway.

"Is this your father, Andrés?"

"My mother." He takes the photo back from me, though he does not seem at all put out by my mistake.

Today is Alejandro's turn to get a gift. Purple cellophane and a ribbon wrapped around a piece of cardboard, under the cellophane a small collection of metal knives and forks.

"Thank you, Andrés, thank you." Without opening it, Alejandro props the package up on display atop the filing cabinet.

And later, after lunch, poor Miguel Ángel arrives. The second specialist, who he saw today, had nothing to add about the swelling in his jaw. But then Alejandro places a call to someone else and they confer, and the decision is made that they will begin radiation on the growth this afternoon. So off Miguel Ángel trundles to Radiation, carrying an order marked *Urgente*. Half an hour later he returns with the news that he has been given an appointment eight days away. Alejandro makes another call and gets the appointment moved up to Thursday, three days from now.

José Manuel writes out a work excuse for Miguel Ángel covering the whole time of the radiation treatment because, as he tells him, "You won't be feeling completely well while this is going on." Otherwise, no one can do very much for Miguel Ángel at the moment. He is nervous, deflated. He had been hoping, as he says, for *something* to begin today. José Manuel and Elsa make a big deal over his white patent leather loafers. Where did those come from? I've never seen shoes like that. They're really pretty. Did you get them in Miami? Yes, he did, he says.

And then, in turn, Miguel Ángel has compliments for me. "Do you have children, Carlitos? No? But you should have some. Any children of yours would be so handsome."

Elsa winks at me and laughs, because these are precisely the same things she herself was telling me a couple of hours ago.

On the weekend José Manuel learned that a gay doctor who works in one of the towns near Wakax saw two of the young men from there, friends of his, and, because they seemed so depressed, he took them off to the coastal island of Holbox for what José Manuel calls an *orgifiesta*.

"These are the guys who are VIH?" I ask.

José Manuel nods. "They stayed until they were fucked out. I spoke with them, too, and when it came to whether they had been using condoms or not they were completely evasive with me."

He is silent a minute, looking away. Then he says, "Sometimes it gets me down, Carter. This morning I had to give a positive result to a seventeen-year-old boy."

Soon after, Russell returns from the end of his day's clinic. He checks to see if there's water in the pot, plugs it in, and plops down in José Manuel's chair. He shows off the new coffee cup he got when he attended a medical conference in Acapulco. The decoration encircling the cup is a color photo montage of the backs of lithe, tanned girls all wearing *tangas*, string bikinis that disappear into the cleft between their buttocks. "I don't know," Russell says. "No, I don't think so." He squirms his own butt around in his chair. "I don't think I'd like something *pulling* all up in there like that."

Then, after the coffee is ready, he says, "Was that boy Andrés in here today?"

Alejandro says, "He was. What about him?"

"I'm no longer sure how much Andrés is really with us—or should I say, I'm not sure that he isn't telling us that he's not going to be around much longer."

"You mean bringing in the photographs for us to see?"

"That, and also— Has anyone else been receiving gifts?"

"There's mine. He brought it today." Alejandro takes down the cellophane-wrapped knives and forks and places them before Russell. "Probably tomorrow his father will come complaining that they don't have anything left in the house to eat their dinner with."

Russell regards the cellophane package, turns it over, lays it back on José Manuel's desk. "It's the impulse to generosity, isn't it? No matter what form it takes." He shakes his head and sighs. "You know, to do this practice, really do it, I would need a lot more heart than what I have. Me, I'm a coward."

POSTSCRIPT: LAS COSAS DE YUCATÁN

DECEMBER 1992–JANUARY 1993

I was back in Mérida the week before Christmas, but only for two days. Almost as soon as Alejandro and I sat down to talk, it became clear that the signs he and I had both interpreted as being mixed had, in fact, been all bad. In the fall a team had come from IMSS in Mexico City to assess the work of the Oficina de Actividades Contra SIDA. Their conclusion was that most of the "regular" treatment—meaning the treatment given the ambulatory patients Russell and José Manuel were dealing with—should be distributed among the IMSS level-one clinics that focus on family and preventive medicine and that only "serious" cases ought to be dealt with at a specialty hospital like the T-1. One advantage to this new "horizontal integration," as they called it, would be to give the general practitioners, disease control, and internal medicine people more familiarity with SIDA. Before the new plan could take effect, the assessors said, Alejandro's group would have to train the level-one doctors in clinical aspects of the disease.

Alejandro had argued that the problem with the new organizational scheme was that VIH-positive patients clearly need special attention from the beginning. Not only are many of their problems difficult to diagnose, but even the "ordinary" ones can spiral off suddenly into a series of dangerous complications. He also explained to the panel from the D.F. that his clinic's use of retrovir was by now a fairly long-term experiment, and that a useful set of data had been collected. Even if the patients who were less ill were sent elsewhere, the T-1 would still need to monitor all the people taking the antivirals.

Initially, the assessors seemed to agree with the monitoring idea. But his other rationales for keeping the clinic together had made less of an impression on them.

I asked what had become of Laura, beautiful Laura with the intransigent husband.

Without access to the expensive medication, Alejandro said, Laura had been unable to get rid of the thrush in her throat. It had grown much worse, and Alejandro had just admitted her to the T-1. As an inpatient she could at least finally get the right drug. But something had happened with the IV they had her on, and now Laura's arm was badly swollen. Alejandro was hoping he could discharge her from the T-1 in time to spend Christmas Eve with her little boy.

José Luis Matú claimed he had taken his jewelry with him when he went to Los Angeles in the fall and had given it all away to friends there. But he appeared for lunch wearing leather and silver bracelets and a silver pin with a North American Indian in a headdress.

"Are those rhinestones?" I asked.

"No, honey, these are diamonds, of course."

The waiter, a stocky Mayan gentleman, stood waiting for Matú to make up his mind. "Tuna?" Matú said. "No—," with a look at the waiter, "I've eaten too much tuna," which cracked the waiter up.

To me in English, "You get that, Charlie?"

"Sure," I said, although in fact I didn't at all.

Matú had information on his friend Miguel Ángel, the "boy" (he was thirty-two) who worked at the T-1 and whose jaw had been so grotesquely swollen in September. Gone. For a while the chemotherapy had worked, Matú said, the swelling had gone down. To keep Matú from worrying while he was in Los Angeles, Miguel Ángel had lied and told him they'd given him an operation and had cut the whole thing away, and that you couldn't see the incision because the stitches were on the inside. But the cancer had metastasized and Miguel Ángel died of a blockage to his heart. Matú had called when he returned from California and was told that Miguel Ángel was in the hospital. When he called there, planning to go and see him, he was told that Miguel Ángel had died. "That was OK, though," Matú told me, "because we had said good-bye before I went to the States."

Then, a moment later, "Such class he had, Charlie. All those little suspenders? He left them for me."

But on the other hand, Héctor, the son of the cantina owner, the patient who was going to be the first SIDA autopsy, did not die when they thought he would. According to Matú, he was up and about and had put on some weight.

In January Alejandro and José Manuel were moved to a new, smaller, less conspicuous office. It took a while for their new phone extension to begin working, and some of the switchboard operators seemed not to have heard of a SIDA clinic at the T-1. Then in February, when I called from California, Alejandro and José Manuel informed me that their new number would be good only through the week because their entire operation was being dismantled. The doctor in charge of one service at the T-1 told Alejandro, "You know, I have nothing in the world against José Manuel personally, but he's made that outfit of yours into a *jaula de locas* (a playpen for queens; also the Spanish title for the film *La Cage aux Folles*)." José Manuel was sent back to the Juárez Hospital, the place he had been drummed out of when they discovered he was VIH-positive. He worked first in orthopedics, and now has become administrator of the emergency room on the afternoon shift. His *muchachos*, as he calls his former patients, come around to see him, but they don't always seem to understand that he's not free to work with them as he was before. Russell continues to see SIDA patients at the T-1 and has been given new duties as well. Alejandro doesn't have an office of his own at the moment, and has had to use some ingenuity to find a place for the records he's accumulated of his work over the last four years. One box of files has gone to the hospital archive, another is stashed out of the way in a corner of a friend's office.

What may have happened is that the SIDA effort at the T-1 succeeded too well. Alejandro is justifiably proud of one of his graphs, which shows the percentage of asymptomatic VIH-positive clients steadily increasing and the percentage of acute cases declining over the years the clinic was in operation. For a variety of reasons, and at a cost, patients in 1992 were living significantly longer and in much better health than they had been in 1989. Alejandro's own politics allow him to see people who are capable of working as "productive" or valuable. To many of his colleagues, unfortunately, the existence of the VIH virus in a person remains proof of a life led irregularly and immorally. To *encourage* such people to use the facilities of an IMSS hospital in order to fight to maintain their health, as Alejandro and his colleagues did, becomes in itself immoral. The Oficina de Actividades Contra SIDA was established in an earlier administration. Though they knew then that the numbers would increase, perhaps they also believed that Dr. Guerrero would somehow manage to "contain" the problem. Instead, in terms of resources needed, he made it grow. And in terms of public perception, he kept trying to make SIDA more visible rather than less.

I know the dangers inherent in accepting the wisdom of cab drivers, but I was taken with the words of Miguel, who drove me to the airport for an early flight the morning of the Solstice. At 6:30 A.M. the sun was only weakly risen, the streets in the center of Mérida were still deserted, everything pastel and covered with a light mist. Miguel was my age, big nose, little mustache. We talked about the pollution. Thinking of José Luis Matú, I pointed out they should at least close 60th Street all the time, the way it is on Sunday, and get the smoky buses out of the center of town. Miguel pretended to agree with me, but he didn't think it would happen. "You know how the politicians think," he said.

"No, how?"

"They think, 'Things in Yucatán should stay as they are.' "

Las cosas de Yucatán deben quedar como están.

NOTES

2. *The Captain's Touch*

1. Some of this research must still have been in progress at the time Dr. Góngora-Biachi and I first talked two weeks before Christmas 1988. Results that he and his associates published two years later (Renán A. Góngora-Biachi and Pedro González-Martínez, "La dinámica epidemiológica") offer a somewhat different set of figures than the ones the doctor gave me. The group of adult male homosexuals referred to here is 124 individuals, not 61, and it is 84 percent of *them* who "prefer" as casual partners boys and young men fifteen to twenty-five years old. Of the 354 male students ages fourteen to twenty-two surveyed in Mérida *preparatorios* or high schools, 51 percent found male homosexuality an "acceptable" phenomenon, and 28 percent found it unacceptable. They estimated that, on average, 30 percent of their comrades had had sex with another male at least once. Twenty-nine percent said they themselves had been invited to have sex with men, but only 5 percent said they had actually participated. (The fuller version of the high school study became the 1992 medical thesis of William Martín Díaz Basto; another of Góngora-Biachi's students, Karla Uribe, evoked a surprisingly similar disparity from Mayan village fishermen on the issue of invitation versus participation in homosexual activity. See pages 116–17 in this chapter.)

2. Morris Steggerda, *Maya Indians of Yucatán*, p. 236.

3. Góngora-Biachi and González-Martínez, "La dinámica epidemiológica," p. 59.

4. Ibid.

5. Zimbrón Levy, *Nuevos enfoques sobre la homosexualidad*, p. 19.

6. Zimbrón Levy, *Nuevos enfoques*, p. 41.

7. John Borrego, "Mexico's Integration and Development Within Global Capitalism," p. 20.

8. Landa, *Relación de las cosas de Yucatan*, p. 124.

9. T.W.F. Gann and J. E. Thompson, *The History of the Maya: From the Earliest Times to the Present Day* (New York: Scribner's, 1931), p. 229, quoted in Steggerda, *Maya Indians of Yucatán*, p. 51.

10. Irwin Press, *Tradition and Adaptation*, p. 101.

11. Walter L. Williams, *The Spirit and the Flesh*, p. 145.

12. Ibid.

13. Ibid., pp. 145–46.

14. Ibid., pp. 146–47.

15. Victoria R. Bricker, *Ritual Humor*, p. 149. Good material can also be found in Gary H. Gossen, *Chamulas in the World of the Sun*.

16. Bricker, *Ritual Humor*, pp. 185–87.

17. Even some of the anthropologists who did know Maya made a point of not listening to this sort of talk. Traveling in the jungles of Quintana Roo in the winter of 1932–33, Alfonso Villa Rojas, the Mérida-born school teacher who became Robert Redfield's assistant and then an anthropologist himself, noted that when the men left the village for a few days, the women became "loquacious," "smiling, bold and coarse in speech. [. . .] in their conversation they do not hesitate to speak quite often of the sexual act in its various aspects. Of course I do not encourage them in talking along those lines" (Villa Rojas unpublished fieldnotes, quoted in Sullivan, *Unfinished Conversations*, p. 41). The women Mary Elmendorf interviewed in Spanish in Chan Kom forty years later were reluctant to talk with her about sex. Yet, when they were gossiping in Maya, Elmendorf says, even without knowing the language she could tell that they seemed to talk about little else (Mary Elmendorf, *Nine Mayan Women*, p. 96).

18. William F. Hanks, *Referential Practice*, p. 122. *Baášal t'aàn*, which is "play speech" or "joking," according to Hanks, depends on a set of words and phrases with double meanings, including the verbs *to take* and *to carry*, which also mean to be sexually penetrated; the word for a "load," which is also a word for genitals; "firewood," a word for erect penis; "honey," for semen; "cheese," for female genitalia; and "tarantula," for vagina (pp. 119–22).

19. Barbara E. Holmes, *Women and Yucatec Kinship*, p. 351.

20. Elmendorf, *Nine Mayan Women*.

21. Gilberto Balam Pereira, a doctor who practiced for a number of years in Valladolid, takes as an index of the effectiveness of midwives the fact that the mortality rate for women in childbirth in village Yucatán is low (0.5 per thousand) (Gilberto Balam Pereira, *Cosmogonía y uso actual de las plantas medicinales de Yucatán*, pp. 90–91).

SUGGESTED READING

Abreu Gómez, Ermilo. *Canek: Historia y leyenda de un heroe maya.* 20th ed. Mexico: Ediciones Oasis, 1969. Translated by Mario L. Dávila and Carter Wilson as *Canek: History and Legend of a Mayan Hero.* Berkeley: University of California Press, 1979.

Almaguér, Tomás. "Chicano Men: A Cartography of Homosexual Identity and Behavior." In *Differences: A Journal of Feminist Cultural Studies* 3, no. 2 (summer 1991): 75–100.

Balam Pereira, Gilberto. *Cosmogonía y uso actual de las plantas medicinales de Yucatán.* Mérida: Ediciones de la Universidad de Yucatán, 1992.

Barrera Vásquez, Alfredo et al. *Diccionario Maya Cordemex.* Mérida: Ediciones Cordemex, 1980.

Bartolome, Miguel Alberto. *La dinámica social de los Mayas de Yucatán: Pasado y presente de la situación colonial.* Mexico: Instituto Nacional Indigenista, 1988.

Bateson, Mary Catherine and Richard Goldsby. *Thinking AIDS: The Social Response to the Biological Threat.* Reading, Mass.: Addison-Wesley, 1988.

Borrego, John. "Mexico's Integration and Development Within Global Capitalism." Unpublished manuscript, 1993.

Bricker, Victoria R. *Ritual Humor in Highland Chiapas.* Austin: University of Texas Press, 1973.

——. *The Indian Christ, the Indian King, the Historical Substrate of Maya Myth and Ritual.* Austin: University of Texas Press, 1981.

Burns, Allan F. *An Epoch of Miracles: Oral Literature of the Yucatec Maya.* Austin: University of Texas Press, 1983.

Carrier, Joseph M. "Gay Liberation and Coming Out in Mexico." In Gilbert Herdt, ed., *Gay and Lesbian Youth*, pp. 225–52. New York: Haworth, 1989.

——. "Participants in Urban Mexican Male Homosexual Encounters." *Archives of Sexual Behavior* 1, no. 4 (1971).

——. *Urban Mexican Male Homosexual Encounters: An Analysis of Participants and Coping Strategies.* Ph.D. dissertation, University of California, Irvine, 1972.

Carrier, Joseph M. and J. Raúl Magaña. "Use of Ethnosexual Data on Men of Mexican Origin for HIV/AIDS Prevention Programs." In Gilbert Herdt and Shirley Lindenbaum, eds., *The Time of AIDS, Social Analysis, Theory, and Method*, pp. 243–58. Newbury Park, Calif.: Sage, 1992.

Delany, Samuel R. "Street Talk/Straight Talk." In *Differences: A Journal of Feminist Cultural Studies* 3, no. 2 (summer 1991): 21–38.

Díaz Basto, William Martín. *Evaluacion de los conocimientos de Inmunodeficiencia Adquirida (SIDA) en una poblacion de estudiantes de nivel medio superior.* MD thesis, Universidad Autonoma de Yucatán, Mérida, 1992.

Elmendorf, Mary. *Nine Mayan Women: A Village Faces Change.* Cambridge, Mass.: Schenkman, 1976.

Everton, MacDuff. *The Modern Maya: A Culture in Transition.* Albuquerque: University of New Mexico Press, 1991.

Galván Díaz, Francisco, ed. *El SIDA en México: Los efectos sociales.* Mexico: Ediciones de Cultura Popular, 1988.

——. "Emprende el Ayuntamiento de Mérida una campaña de moralización social." *La Jornada*, 9 February 1991.

Gmünder, Bruno and John D. Stamford, eds. *Spartacus '90/91: Guide for Gay Men.* 19th ed. Berlin: Brüno Gmunder Verlag, 1990.

Góngora-Biachi, Renán A. and Pedro González-Martínez. "Anticuerpos contra el Virus de Inmunodeficiencia Humana (VIH) en una poblacion de prostitutas de Mérida, Yucatán, Mexico." *La Revista de Investigación Clínica* (Mexico) 39 (1987): 305–6.

——. "La dinámica epidemiológica de la infección por el VIH-1 en Yucatán (1983–1989)." *Revista Biomed* 1, no. 2 (April–June 1990): 53–59.

Góngora-Biachi, Renán A., Pedro González-Martínez, Azeneth Reyes-Pinto, Dora Lara-Perera, Adda López-Peraza, and Gilberto Medina-Escobedo. "Prevalencia de anticuerpos contra el Virus de la Inmunodeficiencia Humana (AC-VIH) y su expresión clínica en un grupo homosexual del sexo masculino de Mérida, Yucatán." *Salud Publica de Mexico* 29 (1987): 474–80.

Gossen, Gary H. *Chamulas in the World of the Sun: Time and Space in a Maya Oral Tradition.* Cambridge, Mass.: Harvard University Press, 1974.

Gray, Francine du Plessix. *Divine Disobedience: Profiles in Catholic Radicalism.* New York: Knopf, 1970.

Guerra, Francisco. *The Pre-Columbian Mind.* London: Seminar, 1971.
Guerrero Flores, Alejandro. "La prueba de anticuerpos VIH, un auxiliar diagnóstico de tipo biológico para un complejo problem de salud, incluso biologico." *Boletin Medico IMSS* (Yucatán) 1, no. 3 (July–September 1991): 16–21.
——. "Factores biopsicosociales asociados con el riesgo de exposición al VIH en personas con antecedentes transmitidas sexualmente (ETS)." Unpublished manuscript, 1993.
Hanks, William F. *Referential Practice, Language, and Lived Space Among the Maya.* Chicago: University of Chicago Press, 1990.
Herdt, Gilbert, ed. *Gay and Lesbian Youth.* New York: Haworth, 1989.
Herdt, Gilbert and Shirley Lindenbaum, eds. *The Time of AIDS: Social Analysis, Theory, and Method.* Newbury Park, Calif.: Sage, 1992.
Holmes, Barbara E. *Women and Yucatec Kinship.* Ph.D. dissertation, Tulane University, New Orleans, 1978.
Instituto Mexicano de Seguro Social, *Ley del Seguro Social.* Mexico: Secrataria General, Jefetura de Publicaciones, IMSS, 1985.
Instituto Nacional de Diagnostico y Referencia Epidemiologicos. *Boletin Mensual de SIDA/ETS* (Mexico) 6 (June 1992): 2192–213.
Landa, Friar Diego de. *Relación de las cosas de Yucatan, 1566.* Translated, edited, and with notes by Alfred M. Tozzer. Cambridge, Mass.: Peabody Museum, 1941.
LeVine, Sarah Ethel, F. Medardo Tapia Uribe, and Patricia Velasco. "Literacy and Knowledge of *AIDS* Among Urban Women in Chiapas, Mexico." Unpublished manuscript, 1989.
Lumsden, Ian. *Homosexuality and the State in Mexico.* Mexico: Colectivo Sol, 1991.
Martínez, Ernesto. *Guía legal del homosexual urbano.* Mexico: EDAMEX, 1985.
Medíz Bolio, Antonio. *A la sombra de mi ceiba.* Mérida: Producción Editorial Dante, 1987.
Mejía, Max. "SIDA: Historias extraordinarias del siglo XX." In Francisco Galván Díaz, ed., *El SIDA en México: Los efectos sociales*, pp. 17–57. Mexico: Ediciones de Cultura Popular, 1988.
Niles, Daniel. *AIDS in Yucatán.* Senior thesis, University of California, Santa Cruz, 1994.
Olson, Charles. *Mayan Letters.* London: Jonathan Cape, 1968.
Ortega Canto, Judith. *Henequén y salud.* Mérida: Ediciones de la Universidad de Yucatán, 1987.
Parker, Richard G. "Sexual Diversity, Cultural Analysis, and AIDS Education in Brazil." In Gilbert Herdt and Shirley Lindenbaum, eds., *The Time of AIDS, Social Analysis, Theory, and Method*, pp. 225–42. Newbury Park, Calif.: Sage, 1992.
——. *Bodies, Pleasures, and Passions: Sexual Culture in Contemporary Brazil.* Boston: Beacon, 1991.

Poniatowska, Elena. *La noche de Tlatelolco: Testimonios de historia oral.* Mexico: Ediciones ERA, 1971. Translated by Helen R. Hunt as *Massacre in Mexico*. New York: Viking, 1975.

Press, Irwin. *Tradition and Adaptation: Life in a Modern Yucatec Mayan Village*. Westport, Conn.: Greenwood, 1975.

Redfield, Robert. *The Folk Culture of Yucatan.* Chicago: University of Chicago Press, 1941.

——. *A Village That Chose Progress: Chan Kom Revisited.* Chicago: University of Chicago Press, 1950.

Redfield, Robert and Alfonso Villa Rojas. *Chan Kom: A Maya Village*, abridged ed. Chicago: University of Chicago Press, 1950.

Reed, Nelson. *The Caste War of Yucatan.* Stanford: Stanford University Press, 1964.

Sepulveda Amor, Jaime et al. *SIDA: Ciencia y sociedad en Mexico.* Mexico: Fonda de Cultura Economica, 1989.

Steggerda, Morris. *Maya Indians of Yucatán.* Washington, D.C.: Carnegie Institution, 1941.

Sullivan, Paul. *Unfinished Conversations.* New York: Knopf, 1989.

Taylor, C. L. "Mexican Male Homosexual Interaction in Public Contexts." In Evelyn Blackwood, ed., *The Many Faces of Homosexuality*, pp. 117–36. New York: Harrington Park, 1986.

——. *El Ambiente: Mexican Male Homosexual Social Life.* Ph.D. dissertation, University of California, Berkeley, 1978.

Uribe Martínez, Karla Beatriz. *Conocimiento de una comunidad pesquera ante el problema del SIDA.* MD thesis, Universidad Autonoma de Yucatán, Mérida, 1989.

Villa Rojas, Alfonso. *The Maya of East Central Quintana Roo.* Washington, D.C.: Carnegie Institution, 1945.

Williams, Walter L. *The Spirit and the Flesh: Sexual Diversity in American Indian Culture.* Boston: Beacon, 1986.

Zimbrón Levy, Ricardo. *Nuevos enfoques sobre la homosexualidad.* Privately printed, Mérida, 1989.

Designer: Teresa Bonner
Text: Sabon
Compositior: Columbia University Press
Printer: Edwards Brothers
Binder: Edwards Brothers